THE STUDENT NURSE

THE
STUDENT NURSE
in the Diploma School of Nursing

By GEORGE PSATHAS, Ph.D.

 Springer Science+Business Media, LLC

ISBN 978-3-662-39248-5   ISBN 978-3-662-40263-4 (eBook)
DOI 10.1007/978-3-662-40263-4

Copyright © 1968

SPRINGER SCIENCE+BUSINESS MEDIA NEW YORK

Ursprünglich erschienen bei Springer Publishing Company, Inc. 1968
Softcover reprint of the hardcover 1st edition 1968

Library of Congress Catalog Card Number: 68-21144

TO IRMA

. . . who helped more than she knows

Preface

The continuing growth of the professions in American society has brought with it an extended and deepened interest in the purposes, substance, and organization of professional education, for it is plainly in the professional school that the outlook and values, as well as the skills and knowledge, of practitioners are first shaped by the profession.
[Preface, p. vii, *The Student Physician,* Merton, R. K. *et al,* (Ed.) , Harvard University Press, 1957.]

Nursing has not yet achieved a professional status comparable to that of medicine, but the leaders of the nursing profession are actively involved in a move toward professionalization. Changes in this direction are being pressed and the struggle to attain professional status within the community of health and medical services and society in general is proceeding with dramatic thrust.

Existing Nursing Education Programs

Within nursing education several different programs exist. Some reflect older, more traditional apprenticeship-in-nursing training philosophies; others represent academic and scientific approaches that aim not only to produce highly skilled practitioners of nursing but nurses who qualify as research scientists. The latter programs are self-consciously concerned with defining the discipline and establishing its claim to a distinctive body of knowledge and skills so that its full claim to professional status can be validated. Ferment, change and controversy characterize nursing education today. New patterns of nursing education are emerging. That professional status can be achieved is doubtful only to skeptics, but that the process of achieving new goals will be long and difficult is acknowledged by all.

Three distinctly different types of schools and patterns of nursing education programs exist today. The collegiate or degree program is university or college-affiliated, shares some core curriculum with undergraduate programs in general, and is moving increasingly toward an academic-scientific orientation in its ideology. Students with the bachelor's degree from such programs are eligible to continue their formal education in graduate schools. Since such programs reduce the hours of clinical experience in hospital wards, their students come to resemble other undergraduates involved in pre-professional training.

The most recently developed program, the associate degree program, prepares students for nursing practice in two years. Less academic work and clinical experience are provided, no degree other than the junior college associate of arts degree is awarded, and continuation into graduate work without additional undergraduate work is not possible. The guiding philosophy of such programs is that nursing is a practical art which can be learned in clinical practice. The junior college concentrates mainly on the basic grounding in academic and theoretical subjects. Most of the clinical knowledge is acquired after the graduate begins to work.

The more traditional and largest in terms of enrollment and number of programs (in 1965) is the hospital-based diploma school of nursing. These three-year programs have begun to include more academic work (some have even affiliated with local colleges or junior colleges to provide instruction in the biological and social sciences) with fewer hours spent in clinical experience in order to reduce the often repetitive aspects of practice that do not necessarily contribute to learning. The diploma school has encouraged its students to seek advanced degrees, while at the same time retaining its more traditional orientation toward recruiting nurses for its parent hospital. The school has been, after all, a hospital school—owned and run by the hospital which usually gives it its name. Some of these schools have been found to be wanting in the level of academic preparation they provide their students.

The Position of the American Nurses' Association

In 1965, the American Nurses' Association (ANA) voted to adopt an objective outlined in a Position Paper which concluded that, in the future, nursing education was to be concentrated in the baccalaureate and associate degree programs. The diploma school was to be "phased out." The following points sounded a clear call:

Education for those who work in nursing should take place in institutions of learning within the general system of education.

The education for all those who are licensed to practice nursing should take place in institutions of higher education.

Minimum preparation for beginning professional nursing practice at the present time should be a baccalaureate degree education in nursing.

Minimum preparation for beginning technical nursing practice at the present time should be associate degree education in nursing.*

In elaborating these points, the ANA specifically singled out the diploma school as an institution that is slowly "disappearing from the American scene" (p. 8). Such schools would continue to train nurses since the demand for nurses remained high, but it was quite clear that for professional nurses the educational requirement would become graduation from a baccalaureate program, and for technical nurses, graduation from a junior college program.

It was recognized that the transition would take a long time. Facilities and trained personnel to provide education were not available, financial resources would have to be developed and, in many instances, community planning for the type of nursing education program to be retained, revised or newly developed had to be undertaken. The road ahead was understood to be difficult. By 1967, it was apparent that there was no likelihood that diploma schools were going to close or modify their programs overnight. The ANA issued a statement urging community planning for nursing education and restated its goals from the 1965 position paper. However, this statement was tempered somewhat by the realization that the diploma schools would have to continue, for just how long it could not be stated, until the desired new educational patterns were developed.

Within the framework of the ANA Position Paper and the subsequent official ANA-NLN Statement on Community Planning

---

* American Nurses' Association, A Position Paper: Educational Preparation for Nurse Practitioners and Assistants to Nurses, American Nurses' Association, 1965.

for Nursing Education (June, 1966), notable progress has been
scored in limited areas. However, unless there is proper planning
conducted from coast to coast the American public may be deprived of the needed increasing supply of nurses in an era when
health care is a basic right of all Americans.

. . . Today, as one year ago, the majority of the country's nurses
are being prepared by the nation's hospital-conducted diploma
programs. NLN accredited diploma programs should *not* (italics
ours) close until the opportunity for enrollment in either an associate or baccalaureate education program is available to all
qualified potential nursing students.*

Nevertheless, the ANA firmly held to its 1965 position. Its
ideological commitment was reaffirmed by noting that:

. . . it was recognized that the shifting of nursing education would
require a number of years but in the spirit of President Ken-
nedy's inaugural address, ". . . let us begin."†

In what might also be interpreted as an attempt to reassure those
who did not have a baccalaureate education or were currently in a
diploma program during the transitional period that nursing education was entering, the ANA issued an additional statement:

As ANA plans for the future, ANA members are assured that:
1. All registered nurses are and will continue to be eligible for
membership in ANA, the professional association for registered
nurses.
2. There is no change in legal status for the diploma nurse.
Nurses graduated from and now enrolled in state-approved diploma programs are eligible upon graduation to become licensed
as registered nurses.
3. The position paper does not in any way affect what nurses
have already achieved, but rather it focuses on the impending
and long overdue changes in the system of nursing education.‡

---

* American Nurses' Association statement urging Community Planning
for Nursing Education, mimeo, February, 1967.
† Ibid, p. 1.
‡ American Nurses' Association, A Date with the Future, American
Nurses' Association, New York, 1967.

Thus, nurses who were in diploma programs and those who would continue to enroll in these programs in the future until the transition had been accomplished were assured that they would not be "second-class citizens." They would not only be eligible for state licensing as R.N.'s but could also join the professional association for nurses, the ANA.

The Student in the Diploma School

Our study began before the ANA issued its Position Paper, although even in 1962 there were indications that pressure to change the diploma schools would increase. The series of studies reported here began in 1962 and followed one entering class in one diploma school until they graduated in 1965, and then the study continued for one year after graduation. While the study was in progress, few changes were introduced into the school's program. Concern for the future was apparent among the faculty but for the class in school during the study, the data provide a picture of what one hospital-based diploma school was like prior to the introduction of any major organizational or curricular changes.

Our main concern is with the students in the school, their characteristics, their experiences while in school, the changes they undergo and the paths they follow after leaving nursing school. Our perspective is social psychological and sociological. We are interested in studying individuals, student nurses, in a social context—that of the nursing school. Characteristics of the situation, the school and its organization, are also examined but, insofar as possible, these are studied in terms of their impact on the students.

How effective are such schools in producing nurses? Are their graduates likely to become the future leaders of the profession? And what of nursing education in general? What can be learned from the organization of these schools, whether they continue to survive or not, that will be of value in developing new programs of nursing education?

Answers to some of these questions began to emerge as the result of our intensive case study of one class of one diploma school. Repeated measurements of this class, including those who left school for various reasons and did not graduate, made it possible to trace the changes that occurred in the students. Comparative data from other studies have also been included in order to provide some perspective for this study.

We did not set out to evaluate the students' effectiveness in performing as nurses. We did not attempt to develop criteria concerning the quality of nursing role performance. These tasks, while worthwhile, were beyond the scope of our study. We concentrated instead on an intensive analysis of one school and its students to learn what we could about this kind of educational institution and its products.

It is our hope that the results of the studies reported here will be of value to nursing in planning for the future. Therefore, wherever possible, we have included recommendations concerning possible directions of change suggested by our findings.

GEORGE PSATHAS
Associate Professor of Sociology
Department of Sociology and
Research Associate
Social Science Institute

Washington University
Saint Louis, Missouri

January, 1968

Acknowledgments

This study was supported by research grant No. NU-00050 from the United States Public Health Service, Division of Nursing, first awarded in 1962 to Albert F. Wessen and John Stern, Co-Principal Investigators for the project entitled, "Role Differentials and Nursing Ideology." Under their direction, the original plan for data collection and the development of research instruments was developed. The grant was renewed for 1965-67 with George Psathas and Albert F. Wessen as Co-Principal Investigators.

Albert F. Wessen was particularly instrumental in the development of the Role Projective Test described in Chapter 4. John Stern and Daniel V. Caputo, Project Director from 1962-65, were instrumental in directing the inclusion of the Edwards Personal Preference Schedule (EPPS) in the design and the collection of personality test data.

I would like to thank the several research assistants who assisted in the data collection and analysis phases of the research: Marian Chamberlain, JoAnne Schwartz, Anne Smith Anzel, Marilyn Ostroff, Anne Salmon and Sandra Gold. A special expression of gratitude is due Marilyn Frank Price for her unstinting and devoted efforts to the success of the project. She was instrumental in establishing and maintaining rapport with the school of nursing and the students during the early phases of the research and also assured the success of every follow-up effort by her persistent and effective effort.

In addition, several graduate student research assistants made contributions to the analysis and organization of the data reported in various chapters. Jon Plapp contributed to many phases of the research, but particularly to the material presented in Chapter 5, "The Personality of the Student Nurse." Martin Kozloff assisted in bibliographic research and in the preparation of the historical overview of diploma schools of nursing presented in Chapter 2, "Diploma Schools of Nursing in America." Cynthia Krueger, while a graduate research assistant, did the participant observation research reported in Chapter 6, "Small Schools, Rules and Evaluations." She held a research appointment at the Center of Community and Metropolitan Studies of the University of Missouri at St. Louis when this chapter was written and is now on the faculty of the Department of Sociology-Anthropology at Brooklyn College.

The support of the Social Science Institute, David J. Pittman, Director, and the Medical Care Research Center, Rodney M. Coe, Executive Director, is gratefully acknowledged. The research was also supported by grant No. CH-00024, United States Public Health Service, Community Health Facilities Branch.

Computations utilizing the Washington University Computing Facilities were partially supported by National Science Foundation Grant G-22296.

A special acknowledgment of thanks is due Albert F. Wessen who first introduced me to the nursing study. He gave considerable time, effort and encouragement during the entire period of the research in his various capacities as director of the Medical Care Research Center, chairman of the Department of Sociology-Anthropology, and as friend and colleague.

To Daniel V. Caputo, now at the Department of Psychology, Queens College, I owe many thanks for his support, encouragement and friendship. His careful reading of the manuscript and his contribution to the clarification of statistical and data analysis problems was invaluable.

I am also grateful to Alice J. Gill for the great care and attention she has given to typing the several revisions of the manuscript.

To my wife, Irma, who knows that I feel more than I can express, my thanks are but a token.

The General Hospital School of Nursing is not identified in any way in this book other than to say it is associated with a large general hospital in metropolitan St. Louis. Every effort has been made to maintain its anonymity in order to protect the identity of those who willingly and cooperatively provided information about themselves, faculty and students alike, to make this study possible. Because of our desire to protect confidences and maintain anonymity, we are unable to thank publicly the faculty, administrators, and students. Without their helpfulness and cooperation in all stages of the research, this study would never have been completed. We hope that the results of the study will be of benefit to them as well as to nursing education generally. To the extent that this occurs, they can know the satisfaction that comes from contributing to the betterment of nursing and nursing education.

G. P.

Contents

Chapter 1

Diploma Schools of Nursing in America*

A brief description of the history of the diploma school of nursing in the United States is presented with special focus on factors that lead to pressure for change.

The diploma school of nursing in the United States is, according to the stated policy of the American Nurses' Association, slated to disappear. The leaders of professional nursing have adopted a policy which involves the upgrading of academic standards in nursing education. At the same time, society's demand for nurses and the increased use of medical services mean that the diploma schools which, in 1965, accounted for 80% of the total number of nursing students who graduated that year, and furnished 78% of all the nurses in practice, are not about to die quickly.

The reasons for the proposed changes in nursing education can be understood through an examination of the history of such schools in America and through a study of one school in particular. This book reports a study of a large diploma school of nursing located in a metropolitan area in the Midwest. The study covered a period of four years in the 1960's prior to and just as the school began to adapt to pressures for change. Our focus is not on the changes that were undertaken, but rather on the situation as it

---

* This chapter was written in collaboration with Martin Kozloff.

existed before these changes. We wish to describe what the school and its students were like and what the implications of that organization and prevailing practices were for the types of changes that might be expected to occur and which, on the basis of our analysis, may be recommended.

THE FIRST SCHOOLS OF NURSING

Nursing education programs in the United States have always had a connection, in one form or another, with a hospital. As Brown points out, "Hospitals [in the U. S.] had had their origin in the eighteenth century in institutions hastily opened upon the outbreak of epidemics of infectious diseases, or in almshouses that often sheltered indiscriminately the insane, feebleminded, criminals, 'paupers,' and the indigent sick."[1] As to the actual teaching of nurses, it began in one of the first training schools for prospective nurses, the Philadelphia Dispensary, established in 1839, where physicians gave students instruction in obstetrics. Significant for future patterns was the establishment of the Nurse Society in connection with the Dispensary, for the Nurse Society began to 1) employ the nurses who had taken the obstetrical course; 2) instruct prospective nurses; and 3) open a nurses' home and school.

In other hospitals where training for nurses was begun, the course of study was practical and clinical; nurses worked and learned as they worked in the medical, surgical, and maternity wards, and also received lectures offered by physicians connected with the institution.

The first formal schools to be established after the Civil War were organized on the "Nightingale" plan which had been inaugurated at the Florence Nightingale school at St. Thomas' Hospital in London, July, 1860. At St. Thomas', the training period was one year. Trainees lived in a nurses' "home," and wore brown uniforms, white aprons and caps. Satisfactory graduates were registered as "certified nurses." This school, then, set new standards for nurses; they were no longer to be regarded as housemaids.[2]

The essence of the Nightingale plan was the principle of "inde-

---

[1] Brown, Esther Lucile, *Nursing as a Profession*, Russell Sage Foundation, New York, 1936, p. 7.

[2] Bullough, Bonnie and Bullough, Vern L., *The Emergence of Modern Nursing*, Macmillan Company, New York, 1964, pp. 102–103.

pendent support and control under an autonomous board, with provisions for graduate staffing adequate for the instruction and supervision of students as well as for the excellent care of patients."[3] Thus, although these schools were independent they had a working agreement with a hospital. Put another way, the Nightingale conception of the training school for nurses was of an *"educational* institution *independently* endowed and organized."[4]

However, the pattern under which the first influential schools for lay nurses were organized, i.e., with financing by nursing school committees and management by nurse superintendents, was soon destroyed. The reasons noted by various authors were the rising cost of education, the changing pattern of hospital economics, the opposition (of physicians) to higher standards for nurses,[5] the demonstration that nurses could lower the mortality rate in hospitals, and the realization that students could save the hospitals money.[6]

The combination of all of these factors led to a change in the relationship between the school and the hospital in which the school became a department of the hospital. As Frank explains it, "Both hospital authorities and nurse training school directors seemed to have found a solution to their respective problems when the nurses passed over to the hospital administrators the responsibility of financing the training of nurses in exchange for the services rendered by the trainees, by subordinating the nursing school to hospital control and by establishing the school as a department of the hospital on the same basis as other hospital service departments."[7] In other words, the new relationship made the schools a financial asset to the hospitals and contributed to the solution of their major employment problem.

The pattern of nursing education which followed upon the new theory of organization—that student nurses worked for the instruc-

---

[3] Bridgman, Margaret, *Collegiate Education for Nursing,* Russell Sage Foundation, New York, 1953, p. 41.

[4] Committee for the Study of Nursing, *Nursing and Nursing Education in the United States,* Macmillan Company, New York, 1923, p. 193.

[5] Frank, Sister Charles Marie, *Foundations of Nursing,* W. B. Saunders Company, Philadelphia, 1959, p. 169.

[6] Bullough, Bonnie and Bullough, Vern L., *op. cit.,* p. 124.

[7] Frank, Sister Charles Marie, *op. cit.,* p. 170.

tion provided by the hospitals—was one in which: 1) Learning became a trial-and-error process under the rationalization of "apprenticeship." 2) Education was sacrificed for "doing and service," with students working as many as seventy or eighty hours a week at menial tasks. 3) There was little time for teaching and none for study. 4) Teachers were few in number because of the rapid proliferation of hospital schools. 5) The length of the training program was increased to two and then to three years because it assured prolonged student service. 6) Mediocre students could now be accepted and graduated, since mediocre students could satisfy the needs of the hospital. 7) Students generally could be exploited.[8]

In sum, as Frank asserts, "By the turn of the century, schools of nursing had already departed from the Nightingale ideal, if they had ever accepted it, and were being governed by the same materialistic principles that governed management generally. Since the nursing schools had proved their value as a department of service in the hospital, the Nightingale foundations were swept away at the expense of quality in education."[9] Almost every hospital in the country, regardless of size, found it advantageous to start a training school. Hospitals were able to enter the field of nursing education without competition because colleges were either all male or, if they did admit females, did not want to offer nursing courses since such courses did not fit the image of what constituted pure intellectual pursuit. Thus, the hospital, rather than the university, became the institutional framework within which nursing education would grow.[10]

However, with the great proliferation of hospital training schools there came both a shortage of teachers, as mentioned earlier, and a lack of uniformity in the schools' curricula. Training programs were developing, then, with widely varying standards, and the absence of uniform regulations for the licensing of graduates allowed such variations to increase.

---

[8] Bridgman, Margaret, *op. cit.* Brown, Esther Lucile, *Nursing for the Future,* Russell Sage Foundation, 1948, New York. Bullough, Bonnie and Bullough, Vern L., *op. cit.* Bunshaw, Col. Raymond H., A Hospital Commander's Appraisal of Nursing Today and Tomorrow, a paper presented at Nurses Professional In-Service Program, U.S. Army Hospital, Heidelberg, Germany, September, 1964.

[9] Frank, Sister Charles Marie, *op. cit.,* p. 41.

[10] Bullough, Bonnie and Bullough, Vern L., *op. cit.,* p. 140, 164.

For several decades after the linking of nursing education to the hospital, the development of nursing education was determined by hospital needs and policies. However, because nursing was and had been (especially since Nightingale) evolving historically as a profession with an image of itself as something other than merely an arm of the hospital, another set of forces began to influence nursing education—the nursing associations and committees and the nurse educators. The clash of the educators with the hospital administrators started a number of trends which are still vital today.

The Committee for the Study of Nursing Education (1923) was one of the first groups of nursing educators to attack the hospital system and demand change. The committee pointed out the inadequacies of hospital schools by saying that: ". . . the average hospital training school is not organized on such a basis as to conform to the standards accepted *in other educational fields; . . .* the instruction in such schools is frequently casual and uncorrelated; . . . the educational needs and the health and strength of students are frequently sacrificed to practical hospital exigencies. . . ."[11] The Committee said that the future lay with the university school of nursing. ". . . they will furnish a body of leaders who have the fundamental training essential in administrators, teachers and the like," and that *the university school should not only train leaders,* but *"develop and standardize procedures for all other schools . . ."*[12] (italics added).

In response to the criticisms of the nurse educators, several changes occurred. Entrance requirements began to go up, with high-school graduation eventually becoming a nearly universal requirement. Curriculum changes also took place. The number of class hours for academic and theoretical subjects increased and the number of hours of repetitive clinical service to the hospital decreased. Nevertheless, in 1948, one author who has provided leadership for nurses asserted that: "By no conceivable stretch of the imagination can the education provided in the vast majority of some 1,250 schools be conceived of as *professional* education. In spite of improvements that have been made in most schools over the years, it remains apprenticeship training."[13]

Many criticisms of the diploma school curriculum pointed out

---

[11] Committee for the Study of Nursing, *op. cit.,* p. 21.
[12] Committee for the Study of Nursing, *op. cit.,* p. 26.
[13] Brown, Esther Lucile, *op. cit.,* p. 48.

its inadequacies. West, for instance, stated in 1950 that 75% of the diploma schools met the minimum standards in biology and physical science (in contrast to 95% of the collegiate schools); only 20% of the diploma schools met the minimum standards in social science (in contrast to 70% of the collegiate schools); and only 70% of the diploma schools met the minimum standards in medical science, nursing and allied arts (in contrast to 90% of the collegiate schools).[14] Similarly, Laughlin pointed out that one of the glaring weaknesses in the service-oriented hospitals was "the scarcity of courses in the humanities."[15] Summing up the criticisms of nurse educators was Rogers who stated: 1) "Nursing theory is rooted in the broad foundation of knowledge that characterizes the *liberally* educated man." 2) "Curriculum objectives must clearly *differentiate professional* education from technology." 3) "The traditional focus on preparing students to work for agencies is profoundly inappropriate for the future needs of society. Nurse educators must become oriented toward a focus on human beings and the life process." 4) "The synthesis of broad areas concerned with the life process must *replace* the segmented, disease-oriented approach, geared to the memorization of multiple, finite details and technical skills." 5) "Laboratory study is subsidiary to the primary objective of transmitting theories and principles." 6) "*The prevailing concept of nursing as a technology must be replaced by a concept of nursing as a learned discipline.*"[16]

The solution to the problems for "professional education" inherent in the hospital school is seen by many nursing leaders to be the collegiate, baccalaureate, or degree program which is conducted within the institutional framework of a college or university. Thus, the nursing school becomes a part of the college, partaking of its academic traditions, methods and aura. Many nurse educators have felt, and continue to feel, that it is only in this setting that nursing education will achieve a professional image.

---

[14] West, Margaret and Hawkins, Christy, *Nursing Schools at the Mid-Century,* National Committee for the Improvement of Nursing Services, New York, 1950, p. 29.

[15] Laughlin, Hugh D., Education Programs in Service-Centered Hospital Schools, *Nursing Outlook, 4,* May, 1956, pp. 268–271.

[16] Rogers, Martha E., *Educational Revolution in Nursing,* Macmillan, New York, 1961, pp. 24–43.

NEW TRENDS IN THE DIPLOMA SCHOOL

There are several ways to look at the trend toward more degree programs. One way is to view it as an outgrowth of the many criticisms directed at the diploma schools. Fred Davis,[17] on the other hand, offers the view that from the beginning there has been a trend toward the degree program which has, however, been slowed by 1) the universities' early views of nursing as being technical, militaristic, utilitarian, and vocational, thereby disposing them to reject the idea of university schools of nursing, and 2) the early linkage of the hospital with the nursing school. Davis notes that it was only when the diploma schools came under the fire of educators, and the *need* for higher education was legitimitized in the light of medical advance and the expansion of the nurses' role from housework and custodial activities to the utilization of intricate techniques, that the trend toward university education for nurses could assert itself.

The trend itself began in 1899 when a course in hospital economics for graduate nurses was inaugurated at Teachers College, Columbia University. In 1909 the first university-controlled school was begun at the University of Minnesota.[18] Since then the number of undergraduate collegiate programs has been steadily, if slowly, increasing. By 1919 there were nine such programs, and by 1929 there were 32; by 1935 there were 70; by 1957 there were 165; and by 1962 there were 177. We note how slow the trend has been, even in the period before the 1930's when the diploma schools were proliferating. Consequently, the diploma schools still produce most of the nation's nurses.

A phenomenon which has accompanied the slow growth in the number of collegiate programs has been the rapid development of associate degree programs. Between 1957 and 1962 the number of such programs tripled, rising from 28 to 84, while the number of baccalaureate degree programs increased by only 7% (165 to 177).[19]

Statistics show that "While the total number of nurses in active

---

[17] Davis, Fred, *The Nursing Profession: Five Sociological Essays,* John Wiley and Sons, Inc., New York, 1966, pp. 147–148.

[18] *Ibid.,* p. 139.

[19] American Nurses' Association, *Facts about Nursing,* 1964 Edition, New York, p. 93 and p. 105.

practice grew by a little over 50% from 1952 to 1964, the number with at least a baccalaureate degree increased by more than 100%.[20] Even with this large increase in percentage, the actual number of practicing nurses who held a baccalaureate degree in 1964 was only 52,100 as compared with 582,000 diploma school graduates in practice. The consistently slow increase in the number of degree programs has prompted the prediction that these schools will not be able to fulfill the "exploding" needs for nursing services. Davis states that the hope of earlier reformers "that professional nursing will one day become a *wholly* university-based profession" may well be delayed of fulfillment, if not repudiated.[21]

There is much data to substantiate the statement that the number of diploma schools is decreasing, while their enrollments are increasing. In 1953, there were 1,026 programs and in 1962 there were only 883. At the same time the number of students has remained fairly constant, being 26,824 in 1953 and 25,727 in 1962.[22] Moreover, at mid-century, 40% had fewer than fifty students, while in 1962 only 14% had that number. In addition, the mean enrollment in 1949 was 83; in 1961 it was 109.[23]

Several reasons are offered in explanation of this trend toward larger but fewer diploma schools. Bunshaw states that the reduction in hospital work and the upgrading of educational standards (two of the earlier changes already mentioned) have taken students "away from the bedside." The resulting *loss of service* increases the cost of hospital operation, as practical nurses and attendants must be hired to replace the students. Since it cost the hospital $750-$2,000 per year (1964) to train each student, "the trustees and directors of hospitals began to regard the nursing school as a liability rather than a necessity which it had formerly been."[24] Consequently, during recent years many have closed. Cunningham explains that because there is an *uneven* distribution of schools, e.g., three or more in one city, one school may close, knowing that

---

[20] Levine, Eugene and Hudson, Helen M., More Nurses Now Have College Degrees, *Nursing Outlook, 13,* 10, October 1965, pp. 31–34.

[21] Davis, Fred, *op. cit.,* p. 150.

[22] Cunningham, Elizabeth V., *Today's Diploma Schools of Nursing,* National League for Nursing, New York, 1963, p. 5.

[23] *Ibid.,* p. 6.

[24] Bunshaw, Col. Raymond H., *op. cit.,* p. 5.

no prospective student will be deprived of schooling. She notes further that expansion is aided by the fact that the larger the school the less the cost per student and faculty member and predicted that "This trend toward larger and fewer diploma schools may very well continue, since the two most frequent reasons for closing . . . —lack of funds and lack of qualified faculty—are problems that are by no means solved."[25]

The reactions of diploma school administrators to both the arguments of the educators and the trends toward collegiate education are of interest because both factors seem to lead to other changes within the diploma schools. Recognizing the status and prestige orientation of the American Nurses' Association and the need, on the other hand, for more nurses, Sleeper stated, in 1958: "What are we seeking—prestige or sound products; status in educational circles, or respect for a job well done; change for change's sake, or *change in our own programs* which will provide graduate nurses who are better able to fill the health needs today, in 1960, or in 1980?"[26] Moreover, she felt that the diploma school had produced nurses for 83 years and that there was no adequate provision to replace it. Her argument, then, was for modification rather than destruction of the diploma system.

The American Hospital Association, too, stated that the diploma school must be strengthened and expanded. The Association "reaffirms its firm support of hospital schools of nursing and its belief that any program of rational planning for nursing services must recognize that the graduates from hospital schools are, and for the foreseeable future will be, the primary source of professional nurses to meet the needs of the American public."[27] The hospitals, however, are recognized as having some vested interest in the continuation of the diploma schools and their support for collegiate education for nurses has been less than whole-hearted.

In addition to the criticism of nurse educators, two other forces for change have been the felt shortage of nurses and the decrease in the proportion of high-school graduates who enter nursing.

---

[25] Cunningham, Elizabeth V., *op. cit.*, p. 6.

[26] Sleeper, Ruth, A Reaffirmation of Belief in the Diploma School of Nursing, *Nursing Outlook, 6,* 11, November, 1958, pp. 616–619.

[27] American Hospital Association, Statement on Hospital Schools of Nursing, Issued August 1, 1963, in *Nursing Outlook, 12, 3,* March, 1964, p. 53.

Although the demand for nurses is increasing, the proportion of high-school graduates entering nursing had dropped from 6 or 7% in the 1950's to 5% by 1962.[28] Furthermore, the very slow increase in the numbers of baccalaureate and associate degree graduates has meant that they have not been able to satisfy the expanding needs for nursing service in hospitals, not to mention other places in which nurses are employed.

One of the changes that began to appear in the diploma schools, and which may be viewed as a counter-trend or as an adaptation of these schools to the changing situation in nursing education, was the shortened program. For example, Roosevelt Hospital School of Nursing in New York cut its program from three years to two (in 1963), hoping thereby to eventually increase its number of graduates by enrolling larger classes. The directors of this school found that "it is possible to cover the necessary content in two years, that we can turn out adequately prepared *bedside* nurses, that the program is saving in time and money for the students and, at the same time, a greater challenge for both faculty and students."[29]

Another change was proposed by Erickson who suggested "a *merger* of several levels of nursing—practical nursing, diploma graduate nursing, and associate degree graduate nursing—into one level of technical nursing."[30]

Cunningham suggested that enrollments could be increased by 2,500 if marriage and residence policies were liberalized in some 432 schools. She noted that only 40% of the 728 schools included in her study facilitated both the admission and persistence of married students; that in 15% only single students were admitted and kept; and that 50% had different policies concerning the admission of married students or the continuation in the school of students who married before completing the course. Some schools included in the 50% gave qualified answers concerning their policies for married students indicating that no single policy was applicable to every case.[31]

---

[28] American Nurses' Association, *Facts About Nursing* (1962–1963 Edition), New York, p. 90.

[29] Scott, Eileen O. and Roche, Elizabeth J., From a 3- to a 2-Year Diploma Program, *Nursing Outlook, 12,* 12, December, 1964, pp. 24–27.

[30] Erickson, Eva H., Why Nurses Need College Education, *Modern Hospital, 100,* February, 1963, p. 146.

[31] Cunningham, Elizabeth V., *op. cit.,* p. 7.

By 1967, a predominant pattern for diploma schools was to operate within the organizational framework of a hospital, referred to as the "parent institution." The hospital is usually utilized as the laboratory for the major share of the instruction in clinical nursing. Whenever the hospital's facilities are inadequate for this instruction other agencies are utilized. Universities used for general education courses are in this category. All but 20 of the 728 schools Cunningham studied in 1963 affiliated with cooperating agencies for two or more weeks of clinical experiences. The majority utilized at least two such agencies.[32]

College or university faculty are relied upon increasingly to teach basic courses. Two-thirds of the diploma schools still use their own faculties to teach basic sciences, but one-third now rely on junior college or university faculties for such instruction.[33] Social sciences are also frequently taught by "outside" faculty partly as a result of the increase in the number of required hours in communications, the humanities, and ethics, religion and philosophy; in 1957 the median time allotted to all three of these areas was 30 hours; in 1962 it was 73.[34]

A commentary on the strength of the link between the hospital and its school at mid-century is found in the fact that in one-third of the schools studied by West and Hawkins, the directors were appointed by the *hospital* board; in one-third by the *hospital* director; in one-sixth by a committee or school board; and in one-sixth by a religious superior. Furthermore, only 27% of the schools reported having a budget separate from that of the parent hospital.[35]

The major changes that are taking place in the diploma schools of nursing in response to the trend toward professionalization can be summarized as: 1) higher admissions standards; 2) an increased number of academic, liberal arts and basic science courses in the core curriculum; 3) a reduction in the number of hours of clinical experience, i.e., time spent working on the wards, and a reduction in the total number of hours required to be spent in the school (for example, the substitution of a basic 9-month academic year—with holiday and summer vacations—for the 11-month year) ; and 4) a

---

[32] *Ibid.,* pp. 10–15.

[33] Catherine, Sister Marian, Nursing Education, *Hospitals, 36,* April, 1962, pp. 118–120.

[34] Cunningham, Elizabeth V., *op. cit.,* pp. 30–32.

[35] West, Margaret and Hawkins, Christy, *op. cit.,* pp. 11–14.

liberalization of the rules concerning marriage (and pregnancy) for students.

According to leaders of the profession, the situation in nursing education in 1965 was one which demanded a clear statement of goals for the future—goals which would be based on an understanding of the development not only of nursing but of general health and medical service. Changes that had occurred in society, and in medicine and medical care, virtually demanded some revision in nursing education. The American Nurses' Association (ANA) examined the situation and undertook the development of a policy to guide planning for the future. It came out solidly in favor of increased professionalization of nursing, higher educational standards, the recognition of different types of nursing specialists, and efforts toward the elimination of vocationally oriented training as the source of professional nurses.

Changes which were explicitly noted by the ANA study group involved the growth of science and technology and the development of new and more complicated treatment procedures. The professional nurse, it was noted, needed better preparation. Not only was there a complex body of knowledge for her to master but in nursing practice there were increasing opportunities for her to exercise critical independent judgments concerning the care of patients. The professional nurse required education to fit that practice. Among the components of nursing practice, which the ANA statement set forth, were:

. . . the use of clinical nursing judgment in determining, on the basis of patients' reactions, whether the plan for care needs to be maintained or changed. It is knowing when and how to use existing and potential resources to help patients toward recovery and adjustment by mobilizing their own resources . . . sharing responsibility for the health and welfare of those in the community, and participating in programs designed to prevent illness and maintain health. It is coordinating and synchronizing medical and other professional and technical services as these affect patients. It is supervising, teaching, and directing all those who give nursing care.

. . . Professional nursing practice is constant evaluation of the practice itself. It provides an opportunity for increasing self-awareness and personal and professional fulfillment. It is asking questions and seeking answers—the research that adds to the body of theoretical knowledge. It is using this knowledge, as well as other research findings, to improve services to patients and service programs to people. It is collaborating with those in other disciplines in research, in planning and in implementing care. Further, it is transmitting the ever-expanding body of knowledge in nursing to those within the profession and outside of it.

Such practice requires knowledge and skill of high order, theory oriented rather than technique oriented. It requires education which can only be obtained through a rigorous course of study in colleges and universities.[36]

This listing of the characteristics of professional nursing practice leads to the conclusion that the minimum educational preparation for the professional nurse should be a baccalaureate degree in nursing.

However, it was also recognized that the need for nursing service was greater than professionally trained nurses alone could provide. Technically trained nurses who may even be specialists in the use and application of certain technical procedures would be needed. Technical nursing practice was therefore defined as a sub-professional status requiring less training, involving less responsibility in the day-to-day care of patients and conducted under the direction of professional nurse practitioners. Educational preparation for technical nursing was defined by the ANA as requiring "attention to scientific laws and principles," but the major emphasis was on technical competence. Therefore, the minimum education for technical nursing was defined as the associate degree in nursing.

Another level of less theoretically and technically trained nurse practitioners was defined as nurse assistants. Included here were nurses' aides, orderlies, nursing assistants and others with on-the-job training. For these practitioners, "short, intensive pre-service programs in vocational education institutions rather than on-the-job training programs" were recommended. In addition to such preparation, in-service and on-the-job training should be given to

---

[36] American Nurses' Association, Educational Preparation for Nurse Practitioners and Assistants to Nurses: A Position Paper, American Nurses' Association, New York, 1965, p. 6.

train the worker to perform specific tasks *delegated by nurses.*[37]

With three levels of practitioners defined, and the kind and amount of education required for practice at these levels specified, it is clear that the graduate of the baccalaureate program would have the highest status and the greatest responsibilities; these persons would be recognized as the professional nurses. The level of preparation for technical nurses would also increase, and the non-degree-granting technical program could be expected to gradually disappear from the scene. These definitions of nursing education and nursing roles for the future represent ambitious efforts to upgrade nursing generally. How well they will succeed remains to be seen.

In Davis' view,[38] the growth rate in the number of graduates from collegiate schools has not been particularly marked, and even assuming "a constant growth rate of approximately 30% for succeeding 5-year periods (since 1960) . . . it still appears doubtful whether by the mid-1970's, collegiate nurses will account for more than roughly a quarter of professional nurse graduates." Davis feels that the trend will probably be toward an increase in the number of nurses graduating from junior colleges and that this new kind of program will not only contribute to the eventual disappearance of the non-degree-granting diploma program but will also detract from the collegiate programs. Students who complete the associate degree program can be licensed as R. N.'s; they can prepare to enter nursing practice in less time than can hospital or collegiate school students; and they have some semblance of a higher education. Therefore, it is possible that the shift in the near future will be from the diploma school to the junior college in greater numbers than from diploma programs to collegiate programs. The tempering of the "strident denunciations of hospital schools by nursing leaders" is seen by Davis as indicating a recognition that the collegiate program is not about to transform nursing into a wholly university-based profession.

We can now see the emergence of collaborative arrangements between junior colleges and hospital schools which may eventually result in a new pattern for nursing education. The introduction of additional academic and theoretical subjects into the curriculum, the reduction in the number of hours of total training, and the

---

[37] *Ibid.,* p. 9.

[38] Davis, Fred, *op. cit.,* p. 150.

possible discontinuation of dormitory living for students enrolled in the associate degree programs may produce a new form of education which retains some of the features of the diploma program but shifts to the junior college the task of setting and maintaining nursing education standards.

How such modifications will be introduced and what forms they will take cannot be accurately predicted. It appears that the diploma schools, as they once were, are about to undergo tremendous changes and some will probably eventually disappear. But until the transition is completed, there is much to be learned from their recent history that can be of value to those who plan to undertake to bring about changes in the nurse's education. It is with this in mind that the results of the present study are presented. The diploma school may be disappearing but its end is not yet in sight. In the meantime, those schools that continue to exist can revise their programs to the benefit of their students and the nursing profession.

Chapter 2

The General Hospital School of Nursing

The "General Hospital School of Nursing" and the characteristics of the entering freshman class are described. The entering students are found to be optimistic, idealistic, hopeful and naive. They are primarily local girls, fresh out of high school, who have not aspired to a college education. They come primarily from the lower middle and working classes. They seem typical of girls who are not set on an academic or career path—they want to acquire the skills and knowledge that will enable them to practice nursing, then marry and work, if possible.

THE SCHOOL

The General Hospital School of Nursing has shown striking parallels, in its history and development, with the development of diploma schools of nursing throughout America. It was founded at the turn of the century at a time when diploma schools were growing in number (between 1890 and 1910 the number of such schools in America rose from 35 to 1,069).[1] In its early decades, the development of its nursing education program was closely linked with the hospital's policies. The board of directors of the hospital passed on

---

[1] Bridgman, Margaret, *Collegiate Education for Nursing*, Russell Sage Foundation, New York, 1953, p. 42.

16

the school budget, appointed the director of nursing education, and reviewed school policies and procedures. The major aim of the school was to provide trained nurses who would not only, in the course of their training, contribute to the nursing service in the hospital, but who would also, after graduation, enter into full-time employment as graduate nurses.

Increasing concern with the quality of nursing education, which as early as the 1920's caused some educators to emphasize the greater importance of the university schools, led many hospital schools to change their entrance requirements and course curricula. For example, from 1911 to 1918 the proportion of schools requiring applicants to be high-school graduates increased from 24% to 43%.[2] By mid-century, the General Hospital School of Nursing required not only that applicants be graduates of an accredited high school but gave preference to those who ranked in the upper half of the graduating class. They were also required to have earned a minimum of 10 academic units in the areas of English, mathematics, social studies, foreign language, biological and physical sciences.

The curriculum within the school had also changed. Basic science courses, including the social sciences, were not only introduced but, by 1963, were being taught by non-nurse educators drawn from local colleges and universities.

A concomitant reduction in the number of hours spent in clinical practice also occurred. In the late 1950's, the introduction of the clinical-instructor system provided an on-the-ward instructor for the nursing student, thus removing her from the direct supervision and control of the head nurse or other representative of nursing service. This change clearly designated the student nurse on the ward as a student rather than as an apprentice or employee. Despite the separation of nursing education from nursing service and the lessened contribution of students to the everyday performance of nursing activities, the program still required three years to complete and, aside from six annual holidays, covered eleven months of the year.

Sixty years after its founding (and at the time of this study) the organization of the General Hospital School of Nursing showed a pattern similar to that of many diploma schools throughout the

---

[2] Brown, Esther Lucile, *Nursing as a Profession,* Russell Sage Foundation, New York, 1936, p. 25.

country. The offices of director of nursing education and director of nursing service were filled by the same person. (They have since been separated.) The school was under the control of the hospital's board of trustees and was viewed as a dependent unit of the hospital rather than as an autonomous educational institution. An important function of the school was, therefore, the education and training of nurses who would eventually work at General Hospital. All graduating seniors were routinely offered positions in the hospital and though it was not expected that all would accept, if none were to have done so the school would have been regarded as failing to carry out one of its major functions.

As is typical of most diploma schools, General guided, supervised, and regulated its students' activities rather closely. Despite the fact that the faculty believed "a nursing student should have the major responsibility for her education" (with reference to obtaining financial assistance), in all other matters the faculty assumed the "responsibility for selecting students and for planning and directing their learning experiences" (General Hospital School of Nursing Bulletin). This paternalistic, or perhaps it should be called maternalistic, attitude of the faculty toward its students will be noted repeatedly throughout this book.

The academic program, in contrast to the clinical, was concentrated in the first year. According to the students, if one managed to succeed academically in the first year, the next two years would be "easy." However, over one-third of the dropouts from the class studied in this research left after the first year. These dropouts tended not to be academic failures, but usually left for other reasons which are discussed in Chapter 3. Of considerable relevance at this point is a statement from the school bulletin which clearly indicated that a student could be asked to leave at any time and for any number of reasons, whether these reasons were specifically enumerated in any rule book or bulletin or not.

> The faculty reserves the right to terminate the student's enrollment in the school at any time if the student's personality, conduct, health or level of achievement academically or clinically makes it seem inadvisable that she continue in the school.

The scope of the faculty's power was extensive and apparently was not checked by any system of review or appeal procedures nor by an effective student government organization. The nursing student was subject to a system in which rules were made, administered and enforced without her involvement or consent. It was at best a benevolent autocratic system.

Most of the class work was presented in the first year, during which time such subjects as chemistry, anatomy, sociology, psychology, physiology, microbiology, nutrition and fundamentals of nursing were taught. After approximately 11 weeks of classroom instruction, the students were introduced to the clinical areas of nursing. During the second session, i.e., the second 19 weeks of the first year, they worked for 4 credit units in medical-surgical nursing (see Figure 1). In the second and third years, greater emphasis was placed on the performance of the nursing role and the application of principles. In these two years, there was a concentration of apprenticeship or *learning by doing*, in contrast to formal instruction in the classroom. This is not to say that formal instruction did not also occur, but there was a major shift in emphasis.

In the first year, emphasis on academic subjects affects many students adversely. They enter nursing school expecting to be nurses in the sense of caring for patients, and then discover that they must be students and attend classes, listen to lectures, take notes and pass examinations. Some of the subjects that they are taught, such as sociology, psychology and microbiology, do not appear to them to be related to the actual practice of nursing.

Further evidence that the academic aspects of the curriculum are regarded as somehow separate from nursing and are considered less relevant than the clinical aspects is the fact that, in discussions outside of class and in their reading activities, students often show little interest in more extensive reading or in the active exploration of areas in which they have proved to be deficient in course work. The notion that research is a legitimate and worthwhile activity for nurses is not an established part of the ideology. The student's attitude is characteristically one of seeking the practical application of things taught. Instructors who have taught such subjects as sociology to students in these schools have commented on the importance of drawing examples and illustrations from experiences that the nurse encounters, or is likely to encounter, in order to show the "practical" value of sociology; the notion that such subjects might be of theoretic interest or of value in themselves, based on values accepted in the liberal arts tradition, seems to have little currency. This is in sharp contrast with collegiate programs which,

Figure 1. Course of Study

Major Area	Year Taught	Lecture	Lab.	Clinical Conf.	Total
Biological and Physical Sciences					
Anatomy and Physiology	1	48	80		128
Chemistry	1	24	40		64
Microbiology	1	24	40		64
Normal nutrition	1	48			48
Social Sciences					
Psychology	1	48			48
Sociology	1	48			48
Non-Clinical Nursing					
History of nursing	2	32			32
Nursing trends	3	32			32
Clinical Nursing					
Nursing I	1	84	76		160
Nursing II	1,2	32			32
Diet therapy	1,2	16		20	36
Pharmacology	1,2,3	64			64
Medical-surgical nursing & specialties	1,2	204		108	312
Obstetric nursing	2	42		54	96
Operating room technique	2	36		12	48
Community health, outpatient & rehabilitation nursing	2	24		24	48
Advanced medical-surgical nursing	3	48		36	84
Psychiatric nursing	2	88		62	150
Nursing of children	3	72		24	96
Administration of patient care	3	8		24	32
Total class hours		1022	236	364	1622

in the first two years of the curriculum, offer college subjects taught as subject-matter fields in their own right, without specific reference to their relevance for nursing.

In her clinical performance the student is continually supervised, evaluated, and rated, not only by the nurses and supervisors on the wards, but also by her clinical instructor. Such evaluations are pooled by the faculty to determine whether the student is making "satisfactory progress" or "becoming a better nurse." By focusing on specific problems, the faculty can indicate what behaviors the student must change in order to meet the criteria for successful performance. In the development of skills for dealing with patients, other persons such as nurses, supervisors, and instructors become important role models and sources of formal instruction and informal advice.

Peer relationships also provide opportunities for the discussion of lessons learned and the sharing of experiences by those who may have figured out how to get along with patients or other personnel on the ward. Assignment to teams makes the students working partners with others from whom help and assistance in the learning and performance of the nursing role can be obtained. Although the patterning of their work assignments in the hospital does not bring large numbers of students together on the wards, there are opportunities for informal get-togethers after hours.

In off-duty hours, the natural groupings of friends, which may or may not have been fostered or stimulated by working relationships or by the initial dormitory room assignments, flourish.

Considerable variation has been observed in students' off-duty conduct although one major interest common to girls of this age may be said to appear and reappear throughout the school years, i.e., dating and marriage. Off-duty hours provide opportunities for dating but the "dating game" also carries back into the work setting. New interns and residents are the subject of much attention when they first arrive on the wards. Romantic concerns appear repeatedly as important elements in projective stories written by freshman girls (see Chapter 4), while more reality-based concerns appear in the stories written by seniors.

Some friendship and extra-curricular activities represent opportunities for tension release and expression. Some of the informal groups, however, seem "dedicated" to the violation of rules which they perceive as obstacles thrown in the way of the student, rather than as contributing in some way to their growth as nurses. The presence of such deviant groups among the student body reflects the emphasis in small residential educational institutions on the evaluation of total performance and the importance of constantly "being on." Because it provides dormitory facilities which are usually located adjacent to the hospital, the school can maintain close supervision over its students' informal activities. It is difficult for the students to escape supervision or observation by faculty, house mothers, and fellow students. Consequently, patterns of evasion can be expected to develop and to become, for some groups, a challenging activity. In other educational institutions the student can go home or to her room at the end of the day and be a different self in relation to other persons who are neither her instructors nor her professional colleagues. But in nursing school, the demands placed on the individual require that she be either a student, a nurse or a student nurse almost constantly with little respite. This may be one reason why weekends become a time for an exodus from the school. Some go home, some go to friends' homes, and some go to motels to "live it up" over a Saturday night.

THE STUDENTS

The students who were studied intensively in this research project were the 79 girls who entered the General Hospital School · of Nursing in September, 1962, as the class of 1965. They were asked to fill out a detailed questionnaire containing questions about their reasons for entering school, what they expected from nursing, what their family background was, and a variety of other questions designed to determine their social characteristics. They were also contacted several times during their three years in the school in order to obtain follow-up data. All girls who left school were subsequently contacted in the summer of 1965, when they would have been graduating, and interviewed. The girls who graduated were contacted approximately eight months after their graduation in a follow-up study to learn whether they were still in nursing and what their plans were at that time.

The characteristics of the entering students in the fall of 1962 will be described here in order to present a profile of the class. The entering students were recent high-school graduates (87%), although some (11%) had worked full-time for more than six months after high school. Four had also attended college for a year or more before entering school. All were girls between the ages of seventeen and twenty, almost all were white (2% Negro), almost all were Christian (66% Protestant, 25% Catholic and 6% Jewish) and a large proportion came from the local community. Approximately 30% came from outside the St. Louis Metropolitan area.[3] Of those residing in the St. Louis Metropolitan area at the time of entering, 10% came from the city of St. Louis, 32% from St. Louis County, and 29% from other parts of the SMA. Only two persons lived in a state other than Illinois or Missouri. The larger proportion had lived in either a city (59%) or small town (28%) and only 6% had lived on a farm; the remainder, 7%, had lived in some combination of these.

For all of these students, attending nursing school meant moving away from home and living in a dormitory. This was a new experience for 70% of the girls; only 11% had ever lived in a dormitory before. In response to an open-end question concerning their expectations for dormitory living, most of the girls (81%) were optimistic in that they expected to like the esprit de corps, friendliness and companionship that dormitory life would provide. Twenty-five per cent of the respondents could think of nothing about dormitory life that they expected to dislike.

As a group, they were not particularly interested in the academic curriculum nor did they feel confident about their abilities to master it. When asked what they expected to like most about nursing school, the largest percentage (29%) mentioned "direct patient care" activities such as "meeting and helping people, contact with patients, and actual nursing." The matter that was next most frequently mentioned was the opportunity to gain knowledge and experience (15%). The least frequently mentioned (2%) was the chance to apply in practice the theory learned in class.

When asked to indicate what they expected to like least, the most frequently mentioned response (34%) pertained to negative aspects of homework and classes (e.g., "too difficult," "boring") and only 6% mentioned the negative aspects of patient care (e.g., working with the helpless and the hopeless) or unpleasant duties and aspects of work such as hours (9%).

When specifically asked what they expected to be of particular

---

[3] The Metropolitan Area includes the city proper, three counties in Missouri and two in Illinois.

difficulty in nursing school, 50% mentioned studies or lack of confidence in their scholastic abilities. On the other hand, a large percentage (35%) did not think that anything would be particularly difficult for them. Only 1% mentioned the problem of working with the helpless or hopeless and the same small percentage listed personal feelings of inadequacy in practice.

The strong interest of these students in patient care, rather than academic or intellectual challenge, was also manifested in their responses to a check-list of nuring specialties. The areas of specialty were divided into "hospital" and "non-hospital," and the students were asked to indicate their first, second and third choices. In rating the hospital specialties, pediatrics was most often preferred (21%), obstetrics came next (16%) and rehabilitation ranked third (11%). Most students (80%) indicated that they were interested only in hospital specialties and gave no first or second choice of non-hospital specialties. When a non-hospital specialty was mentioned, the most favored first choices, selected by an equal number of respondents, were public health, private duty and industrial nursing; the most favored second choice was nursing education and the most popular third choice was working in a physician's office.

Reasons given for the first choice of specialty were most frequently related to patient characteristics. For example, the student said she loved babies, or that old people were rewarding to work with (25%). The next most frequently mentioned reason involved job characteristics (20%) with such things as the scientific or medical interest of the specialty or the opportunity for the utilization of certain skills which it provided. The third most frequently mentioned reason was a general statement such as "interest" (15%).

Among the reasons for second choice of specialty, patient characteristics were again the most frequently mentioned (18%). Reasons for third choices involved job characteristics as the major consideration (18%), e.g., occupational demand and job security.

It seems then, that these students' choices of specialty were made in terms of patient characteristics, with such factors as job security or the extent to which the job would permit the application of nursing skills being given secondary consideration.

Also relevant here are responses to a question which asked for a listing of three reasons why these girls selected nursing. Almost half of the first-mentioned reasons (49%) could be classified as altruistic. The students stated that they wanted to help people and that they saw nursing as the best means of doing this. Some also mentioned that they could serve God through nursing.

Among the reasons listed as second were factors such as liking the hospital atmosphere, the need for nurses, and the variety and excitement of the work. Mentioned under the third reason for choice of nursing were specific job characteristics including job security (34%).

The reasons given least often by the students were, for first choice, self-interest (e.g., to achieve satisfaction or happiness, to aid personal development, good basis for raising a family, 4%); for second choice, educational objectives such as wanting to get more education, 2%; and for third choice, educational objectives, 1%.

These data indicate that the entering students were not strongly motivated by academic or intellectual interests.[4] One bit of evidence not consistent with this pattern is the fact that almost one-third (31%) had considered teaching as an alternative to nursing and, when asked whether they planned to continue their education after nursing training, 54% responded affirmatively. Of these, 48% planned to work for a B.S. degree. Aside from the responses to these questions concerning alternative occupations considered and plans for further education, there was considerable evidence to indicate that the entering students were not interested in the academic and theoretical side of nursing, but rather had a practical, vocational interest.[5] What they valued was working with people, helping others, and being involved in direct patient care. The

---

[4] Dustan's study, comparing students who entered three types of programs, associate degree, collegiate and diploma, found that the diploma school students have the least scholarly and scientific interests. Dustan, L., Characteristics of Students in Three Types of Nursing Education Programs, *Nursing Research, 13,* 1964, pp. 159–166.

[5] Dustan notes that the students in the three types of programs she studied all shared as reasons for choosing nursing "interest in and liking for people," "interest in caring for the sick," and "interest in the medical field." However, degree students chose their programs because of opportunities for professional advancement and personal development; associate degree students for reasons of expediency (e.g., cost, length of program); and diploma students because it "would provide them with the preparation to do what they wanted to do." Dustan, L., *op. cit.,* p. 166.

challenge of nursing was not seen as an academic-scientific-intellectual enterprise, but rather as an opportunity to provide care for others who are in need of help.

Yet, nursing was perceived as an important commitment involving years of investment in training and the expectation of continuing education and work. Almost all (97%) said that they wanted to continue working as nurses after marriage. They expected to delay marriage until the completion of nursing training. (At the time of entry, school rules did not allow a student to be married until the last five months of her senior year.) Only one respondent mentioned that she planned to marry within three years, which would mean while she was still in school.

These students reported that they had considered entering nursing for a long time. About half said that they first considered nursing before they were in eighth grade and another third while they were in the ninth or tenth grade. The final decision, in contrast to the age at which nursing was first considered, was made before the tenth grade by only about 25% of the respondents and after the eleventh grade by the rest.

Another aspect of commitment to the occupation is indicated in responses to questions concerning alternative occupations that they may have considered. The majority had contemplated entering fields which are traditionally defined as open primarily to women; i.e., teaching, being an airline stewardess or doing clerical and secretarial work. The most frequently mentioned alternative field, teaching, involves a period of training after high school.[6] Being an airline stewardess may have been the alternative chosen by some because of its earlier association with nursing. However, it is more likely that it was chosen because some students are oriented more toward glamour, adventure and excitement in an occupation, not to mention their interest in opportunities to meet eligible young men and to marry.

At the time of entry, none doubted that they would complete

---

[6] McPartland also noted that the most frequent occupational alternative mentioned by diploma school nurses in his study was teaching; next was office work. McPartland, T., *Formal Education and the Process of Professionalization: A Study of Student Nurses*, Community Studies, Kansas City, Missouri, 1957.

the training program, since this is necessary before one can enter practice. Nursing is not like some other kinds of programs, e.g., engineering, which one may leave after partial completion and still obtain a job in the field. Furthermore, 97% stated that they planned to work as nurses after marriage. The ideology of the nursing school stresses a professional orientation such that the student who seriously considers leaving nursing or becoming a nurses' aide is likely to receive little support from her peers or the faculty. Students learn very early that being an aide is not as desirable as being a nurse. If one thinks they are equivalent, it is an indication that one has failed to acquire the attitude toward occupation and self-in-role which are important early learnings in the school.

The family backgrounds of the entering students, judging from fathers' and mothers' education and occupation, were lower middle class or working class. Many fathers (37%) fall into the occupational classification of craftsmen, foremen or operatives. Another large percentage were managers or proprietors (21%) and 10% were in some profession. Of those remaining, 11% were in clerical or sales work, 12% were service workers or laborers and 8% were farmers.[7] None of the fathers were doctors. The education of the fathers reflected this occupational distribution in that 20% had gone to college (14% completed college), 37% had completed only high school and 23% had had some high-school education but had not graduated. Of the remainder, 17% had stopped at the eighth grade. For 2.5% (2 cases) no data were available.

The distribution of the mothers' education showed a similar pattern with a smaller percentage (16%) having gone to college and only 4% having completed college. The largest number (42%) had completed high school, and 19% had had some high school. Of the remainder, 21% had stopped at the eighth grade and 1% had

---

[7] Comparing students in the three types of schools, McPartland found that, judged by father's occupation, students in the collegiate school ranked highest, "those in three-year church-sponsored schools are more likely to rank near the middle and those in three-year public and voluntary schools are more likely to come from families in the lower ranges of social prestige." McPartland, T., *op. cit.*, p. 27. The students in this school are roughly comparable to those in the diploma school studied by McPartland, i.e., in the middle and lower ranges of socioeconomic rank.

not completed elementary school. Considering the mothers' work, 4% had been nurses and an equal number had worked as a medical assistant other than a nurse. Most of the mothers (90%) had worked at some time in their lives and 43% were presently employed. The types of occupations in which they worked reflect the general pattern of women's occupations: professional, 9%; managers or proprietors, 2%; clerical and sales work, 49%; craftswomen or forewomen, 4%; operatives, 11%; and service, 14%. Some 10% had never worked.

Given these characteristics and expectations, students who entered the General Hospital School of Nursing in September, 1962, can be described as optimistic, idealistic, hopeful and naive. In short, they displayed characteristics that any applicant or entrant into a new field would be expected to reveal when answering questions about her attitudes and expectations. There were few negative statements, little indication of anxiety or concern about an ability to "make the grade," and a generally optimistic attitude such as usually accompanies a repeatedly expressed interest in working with and helping people. Nursing is an attractive field and entering students' enthusiasm for it is high. We would not expect that statements made at this time would show any substantial correlation with subsequent behavior since these statements show so little variation.

The entering students were local girls, fresh out of high school, daughters of lower middle- and working-class parents who aspired to enter an occupation which in terms of socioeconomic level would be a step above that of their parents, and who had every intention of staying in school until they completed the course. After graduation, they expected to marry and raise a family but they intended to work as nurses even after marriage. Most were not particularly interested in the academic or theoretical side of nursing but were motivated primarily by a desire to help people. They anticipated some difficulty with academic subjects but nevertheless expected to complete the course and possibly continue to work toward an advanced degree.

They had not aspired to college but set their sights on the diploma school of nursing; they decided to enter nursing while in high school but had considered it as a field for even longer. They seemed typical, in many ways, of girls who do not plan on college and an academic career. They wanted to acquire the skills and knowledge that would enable them to practice nursing, then marry or work. Marriage and work were not seen as incompatible. Becoming a nurse was, for them, an important life goal.

In subsequent chapters we shall see what happened to these girls as they progressed through the nursing school. The reality of school, and the multiple forces which it represented for socialization of the student, produced results which probably neither students nor faculty could have predicted.

Chapter 3

Who Leaves School: The Dropouts

Several approaches to studying the dropouts from General are presented. Intellective predictor variables, such as high school rank, intelligence and aptitude test results, and social characteristics, such as socioeconomic class, show that intellective predictors are neither consistent nor stable predictors of dropping out and that few social characteristics other than the combination of low ability and low social class predict who will drop out.

An analysis of the official reasons for a girl's leaving reveals discrepancies between these reasons and those which the girls themselves acknowledge. Official categories lump together a number of different types under one heading and tend to imply a single factor cause of dropping out. After an intensive examination of individual cases, a new typology is presented. This typology is based on the view that dropping out involves a complex relationship between the individual student and the school. Individual variables are therefore not adequate to predict dropouts. The implications of this new classification for reducing the number of dropouts are discussed.

INTRODUCTION

Despite the care and attention given to the selection of the freshman class at the General Hospital School of Nursing, 37% did not complete the program. The largest proportion of dropouts, 57% (17 out of 30), left during the first year. Another 33% (10) left during the second year, all before the end of the seventh month of the second year. The other 10% (3) left early in the third year. Students who leave after the first year represent the greatest financial loss to the school which, by then, has invested more in their education than it does during either of the other two years. By the second year all major subjects have been passed; clinical training and experience constitutes the bulk of the third year program. Since the reasons for the students' leaving are often not understood by school personnel, it is difficult for the school to take preventive or remedial action to reduce the rate of loss. Findings from other studies, as will be shown in this chapter, offer little hope for an early solution to the problem. Part of the reason for this is that school personnel have an inadequate concept of the dropout syndrome.

Our first effort to understand the dropout problem led us to search the literature for reports of the many studies which have been done on predicting success or failure in nursing school. Despite the many studies reported, the results from the search for predictors of success in school have not been very encouraging. Fishman summarizes research in this field with reference to colleges, as follows:

> A recent review of all of the studies of college guidance and selection completed during the decade 1948–58, both published and unpublished, reveals this area of research as undoubtedly among those most intensively investigated in the entire field of educational research. There are certainly not many other topics that would yield 580 studies within a single decade, many of them formulated fully for use in educational institutions. But what is the upshot of it all? Unfortunately, it can all be summarized briefly. The most usual predictors are high school grades and scores on a standardized measure of scholastic aptitude. The usual criterion is a freshman grade average in college. The average multiple correlation obtained when aiming the usual predictors at the usual criterion is approximately .55. The gain in the multiple correlation upon adding a personality-test score

to one or both of the usual predictors, holding the criterion constant, is usually less than +.05.[1]

A correlation of the order of .60 is not large enough to account for more than 36% of the variance. Thus, two-thirds of the variance remains unexplained. Stated differently, no more than about one-third of the forces related to successful completion of training can be accounted for.

Given the results of the use of intellective predictors, some investigators are increasingly turning to such non-intellective predictors as personality tests, biographical inventories and attitude tests. In fact, it appears as though this will be the "fashionable" trend in research during the next few years. Fishman notes, however, that personality predictors often correlate just as highly with high-school grade average or with the results of scholastic aptitude tests as they do with freshman grade averages in college. Because these instruments have such a large amount of common variance, they do not seem to be measuring something sufficiently different from whatever it is that the usual intellective predictors measure to warrant their use.

The distinction between intellective and non-intellective measures is at best a hazy one, since the common intellective measures covertly measure non-intellective factors as well. The commonly used high-school grade average is not a measure of intellective performance only. It also reflects the degree to which the student adapted to the high school's norms, the degree to which his personality agreed with the model of the preferred personality in that high school, the success with which the student interacted with his teachers, and a host of other non-intellective factors. As Fishman has put it, "high-school grades are, in fact, a summary of a life story." (p. 478) They reveal in a single measure the results of a complex life pattern. It is easy for investigators to be fooled into thinking that because the grade point average is a single score it represents a single phenomenon.

There is a singular lack of theory in the research done thus far using predictive variables. The usual kind of intellective predictor study makes the theoretical assumption that past performance

---

[1] Fishman, J. A., Social Psychological Theory for Selecting and Guiding College Students, *American Journal of Sociology*, *LXVI*, March, 1961, pp. 472–482.

is the best key to understanding future performance and that there is an underlying associational or correlational model which says that past, present and future behavior are somehow related. What is missing is any indication of why such a relationship exists and how it is maintained.

Once again, looking at the high-school average as an example, Fishman notes:

> As things stand, high school average—based as it is on performance over an appreciable time period (and standardized aptitude or achievement tests—intended as they are to equalize the marking scale across high schools) are *both* reflections of the consequences of non-intellective factors in the applicant and in his environment. When we refine our measures of high school performance (whether these measures be grade averages or test scores), we invariably do so by further increasing the degree to which they validly reflect stable non-intellective factors. Thus, test scores or high school averages differentially weighted (e.g., for the previous college performance records of the high school's graduates, for community size, and for the size of the applicant's graduating class) must correlate more with scores on many a non-intellective predictor than will high school averages or test scores that are not so weighted. This must be so because the corrected intellective predictors are being corrected for some of the very factors that many non-intellective predictors are seeking independently to predict." (p. 477) [2]

Thus, the efforts to improve the intellective predictor often result in the inclusion of non-intellective factors. The lack of a theoretical basis for the inclusion of some of these factors remains a significant gap. There can, indeed, be an improvement in prediction, but ways of bringing about such improvement are not clear.

Another point needs to be made. Even if such improved predictors could be discovered and the degree of correlation between predictors and criterion variables improved, an important question concerning the value of their utilization remains. It is quite possible that an unrestricted use of such predictor variables would result in doors being closed to people who might otherwise have entered and successfully completed the program. It is possible to "freeze" the

[2] Fishman, J. A., *ibid.*

educational environment in such a way that only those who are able to adapt to *it* would be selected for admission. An alternative, which such designs neglect, is the revamping of the institution itself to provide programs which can be successfully completed by a variety of applicants. Implicit, therefore, in the use of such predictors for selection is not only the freezing of admissions policies in order to improve productivity but also the likelihood that an institutional rigidity will develop. The institution can argue that it need not modify its own procedures since the applicants selected are all "successful" high-school graduates. Meanwhile, students who would be capable of becoming qualified practitioners in the profession would be excluded because they were judged unable to adapt to the demands of the educational institution. Since these demands may have little to do with the performance required of practitioners after completion of training, it is possible that human values would be sacrificed and that the profession, despite its need for additional members, would suffer losses.

The form of our investigation of dropouts from schools of nursing departs, therefore, from the usual predictive model. It is our contention that a new direction in research on this problem requires examination of the school's procedures after students have been admitted. The thrust of our concern is with the assessment of the school's ability to adapt to the problems presented by its students rather than the student's ability to adapt to the school. We assume that students enter with some degree of interest, motivation, and ability. How is their potential realized, their motivation enhanced, and their interest maximized? Can the school modify its procedures in some way so as to increase the likelihood that more students will graduate? If so, in what direction do such changes have to be made?

To determine why students left before completing the program, we decided to examine the dropouts because we felt that such an examination would reveal something about their characteristics and, in addition, it would reveal important features of the school itself. However, we first undertook an examination of the usual predictor variables to learn whether the degree of correlation between these and outcome criteria was higher or lower than had been reported in the findings of other studies. Some refinements were added in this study to test the assumption found in most research that predictor variables show the same pattern of relationship with the same outcome variables when measured at different times. That is, do high-school grades show equally high correlations with first-year grades that they do with second-year grades in nursing school? Does the outcome, dropping out of school, show the same relationship to intellective predictors whether it occurs in the first or second year? Answers to these questions, we thought, would make a better assessment of the value of predictor variables than had previously been achieved.

After we had assessed the predictor variables, we examined the case histories of the dropouts because we wanted to learn how the school classified these students and what "causes" were imputed to their leaving. Predictor studies generally assume that the individual's characteristics are the major determinants of successful completion of the program. We wanted to learn how the institution viewed the student's behavior and performance and thus shift our focus to those institutional forces that may have been involved in the student's success or failure.

THE PREDICTIVE APPROACH

Our first approach to understanding why students leave school involved the most frequently used procedures in predictive studies.[3] In this way, we hoped to assess the degree to which these predictors would predict for this school and for diploma programs.

Studies of nurses reviewed by Taylor, et al.[4] indicated that the variables which showed high correlations with certain criteria of nursing school performance were IQ tests, aptitude tests, and rank in high-school class. Scores on pre-admission tests and high-school rank were used most often by nursing schools as criteria of selection.[5]

---

[3] This phase of our research is reported more fully in Plapp, J. M., Psathas, G., and Caputo, D. V., Intellective Predictors and Success in Nursing Training, *Educational and Psychological Measurements, XXV*, No. 2, 1965, pp. 565–577.

[4] Taylor, C. W., Nahm, H., Loy, L., Harms, M., Berthold, J., and Wolfer, J. A., *Selection and Recruitment of Nurses and Nursing Students,* Salt Lake City, University of Utah Press, 1963.

[5] Jacobs, J. H., *The Nursing School Applicant,* Careers in Nursing Committee, Special Report No. 5, Philadelphia, Pa., Southeastern Pennsylvania League for Nursing, 1959.

The most frequently studied criteria of success in nursing school have been measures of academic performance and of continuance in school. Grades given in clinical courses (e.g., medical-surgical nursing) have been studied much less frequently than grades in academic or theory courses. Correlations between intellective predictors and clinical performance have been shown to be lower than correlations between intellective predictors and academic performance.[6]

The predictor variables that were available for studying the students in this school were the following: high-school rank (HSR); the 1937 Gamma AM Form of the Otis Quick Scoring Mental Ability Tests (OTIS); and the Nursing Admissions Test of the Scholastic Testing Service (NAT). The latter two tests were administered prior to the students' admission to the school. These variables were considered singly and in combination.

The criterion variables to which these predictors were to be related were successful completion or leaving school by the end of the first year and, separately, leaving in the second year. Grades were another outcome criterion. These were divided into academic and clinical course grades and further divided into first- and fourth-quarter grades of the first year. Academic course grades for the first quarter included those for fundamentals of nursing, chemistry, anatomy and sociology; the sole academic course taken in the fourth quarter was normal nutrition; and the grade for clinical performance in the fourth quarter was that for medical-surgical nursing. Since some students had left before the fourth quarter of the first year, correlations between the predictors and the criteria were computed only for that group of students that had obtained grades on both occasions, i.e., those who completed the fourth quarter. However, correlations were also computed between the predictors and the criterion of first-quarter grades for all students who took the first-quarter examinations including those who later dropped out.*

The number of students who left school in the first year was 17. By the end of the second year, an additional 10 had left. Third year dropouts (3) were not included in this analysis since all of

---

[6] Taylor, et al., op. cit.

* Of the total of 79 students, information was not available on all of the predictors for two, thus reducing the total to 77.

them were forced to leave because school rules did not permit them to marry and remain in school. All were progressing satisfactorily toward the completion of the program. They will be considered in some detail later in this chapter in order to demonstrate how different they were from the first- and second-year dropouts.

Significant correlation coefficients* were obtained (*see* Tables 1 and 2) between each of the predictors and at least one of the criteria of school performance. The only two criteria for which none of the predictors bore a significant relationship were those of dropout status during the second year of school and fourth-quarter academic

Table 1. Correlations between Predictor Variables and
Criterion of Dropping Out of School in First or Second Year

	All Dropouts (27) vs. All Others (50)	First Year Dropouts (17) vs. All Others (50)	Second Year Dropouts (10) vs. All Others (50)
Single Predictor			
OTIS	.11	.20	.06
NAT	.23	.26a	.11
HSR	.22	.30a	.04
Combined Predictors			
OTIS and NAT	.19	.25a	.03
OTIS and HSR	.21	.32a	.01
NAT and HSR	.29a	.35a	.10
OTIS, NAT, and HSR	.25a	.33a	.04

aSignificant at .05 level

grades. In general, correlations between intellective predictors and academic performance were highest in the first year. This pattern strongly suggests that leaving school during the second year is not

* Correlation coefficients computed were point-biserial between each predictor and each criterion. The predictors comprised the continuous, and the criterion the discrete, variables. Grades were divided above and below the median to form discrete variables. Pearson r was used to assess the degree of inter-correlation between the three objective predictor variables.

Table 2.   Correlations between Predictor Variables and
Criterion of Grade Performance by Quarter and
by Academic or Clinical Courses

	1st Quarter Academic All Students N = 77	1st Quarter Academic N = 60[a]	4th Quarter Academic N = 60[a]	4th Quarter Clinical N = 60[a]
Single Predictors				
OTIS	.30[c]	.36[c]	.01	.22
NAT	.27[b]	.25	.12	.28[b]
HSR	.44[c]	.36[c]	.14	.09
Combined Predictors				
OTIS and NAT	.32[c]	.33[c]	.07	.27[b]
OTIS and HSR	.46[c]	.45[c]	.10	.19
NAT and HSR	.45[c]	.39[c]	.17	.24
OTIS, NAT and HSR	.44[c]	.42[c]	.12	.25

[a]First year dropouts (N = 17) are excluded
[b]Significant at .05 level
[c]Significant at .01 level

an "academic matter" but rather that reasons related to motivation, personal factors, and clinical performance become more salient. Given the fact that academic courses are "bunched up" in the first year of school, this finding is not striking. The correlations, though statistically significant, ranged between .25 and .46 with the higher of these accounting for approximately 21% of the variance. Even for that part of the nursing school experience which is primarily academic, intellective predictors do not account for most of the variance. There is not sufficient basis, as these findings show, for placing any greater reliance than already exists on these criteria as screening devices for deciding on admissions into school. Compared with results of studies of college students, these predictors do not show correlations of comparable magnitude.

Combining predictors did not produce any clear advantage over the use of single predictors. The NAT was the only single predictor showing a significant correlation with fourth-quarter clinical grades $(r = .28)$. No single or combined set of predictors showed significant correlations with fourth-quarter academic grades.

Despite the low correlations, the present findings are significant in that intellective factors and dropout status in nursing school are shown to be related for the first year but not for the second. Correlations between predictors and grades were generally higher than correlations between predictors and the criterion of remaining in or leaving school. A possible reason for this lies in the relation between academic and non-academic factors in dropouts. Teal and Fabrizio[7] found that, for all nursing programs, lower percentages of students in the upper third of their high-school class were academic dropouts. For non-academic dropouts, larger percentages were in the upper third and there was an inverse relationship between class standing and non-academic dropout.

We can next consider the assumption of the consistent predictive power of intellective predictors over time. The results show that none of these variables, either singly or combined, shows a consistent correlation with time (first or second year) when the girl dropped out or academic grades (first and fourth quarter). Therefore, intellective predictors that show high correlations with academic performance criteria early in the program (when used as part of a selection battery) may be inappropriate, if not misleading, for use as predictors of subsequent performance. Furthermore, if we can regard performance in clinical courses as closely related to performance in the occupational role, these findings can be interpreted to mean that intellective factors bear little relation to clinical performance.

The girls who left early in the first year may therefore represent a group for whom low ability operates forcefully and early in the program when academic performance is most important. However, among these girls were some who did not rank in the lowest ability group but rather seemed to have personality problems which interfered not only with academic performance but also affected faculty evaluations of their suitability for nursing. Instead of representing a homogeneous group, even on the characteristic of ability, the girls who left early included a variety of types or, in terms of the predictors, a variety of combinations of these variables and others.

Before examining each case in greater detail, we decided to examine such other characteristics as social background and atti-

---

[7] Teal, G. E. and Fabrizio, R. A., *Causes of Student Withdrawal From Nurse Training,* Final Report, Public Service Research, Inc., Stamford, Connecticut, n.d.

tudes to determine whether these would distinguish the two groups of successful and unsuccessful students.

First- and second-year dropouts were combined and compared with those who were still in school at the end of two years. Because of the importance of intellective factors, some comparisons controlled for these variables by classifying students according to whether they were above or below the median of the nursing-school class on rank in high-school class* and percentile rank on the Nursing Admissions Test. Those above the median on both criteria were considered to be in the higher ability group and those below on both criteria in the lower. Those who were above the median on one and below on another were placed in a middle category. These will be referred to as ability groups.

The combination of father's occupation and education in the Hollingshead two-factor index of social class[8] reveals a relation between social class, ability level and leaving school (*see* Table 3). Social class statuses were grouped into two categories, high and low. A larger proportion of the Outs than Ins are of lower social class. (19 of 24, 79%, vs. 25 of 47, 53%). Moreover, those who are of a lower social-class level and of low ability are more likely to leave school (10 of 12, 83%) than are those of a higher social class level and low ability (1 of 10, 10%). The combination of low ability and low social class seems doubly difficult to overcome. This is comparable to a finding reported by Ecklund[9] that social class is an important determinant of college graduation for students from

---

* If high-school rank, as reported on a student's entry form, were used, we could not compare one girl with another since girls came from schools of different sizes. Thus, to be 25th in a class of 25 is different from being 25th in a class of 200. Each girl's rank was divided by the size of her graduating class to determine which percentile she was in. The percentile values were then arrayed and rank ordered. Thus, the girl who was in the 97th percentile in her graduating class was the highest ranking person in the entering class in nursing school, whereas the girl who was in the 23rd percentile was the lowest ranked person in the entering class. Incidentally, the highest ranked girl did not complete the program, while the lowest did.

8 Hollingshead, August B. and Redlich, Frederick C., *Social Class and Mental Illness,* John Wiley and Sons, New York, 1958, pp. 398–407.

9 Ecklund, B., Social Class and College Graduation: Some Misconceptions Corrected, *American Journal of Sociology, 70,* 1964, pp. 36–50.

Table 3. Social Class by Ability and Dropout Status

Ability Group	Social Class									
	High I–III			Low IV & V			No Info.		Total	
	Out	In	Total	Out	In	Total	Out	In	Out	In
High + +	1	6	7	3	11	14	1	1	5	18
Medium + −										
− +	3	7	10	6	12	18	1	2	10	21
Low − −	1	9	10	10	2	12	1		12	11
N	5	22	27	19	25	44				
%	19	81	100	43	57	100				

the lower rank of their high-school classes, but relatively unimportant for those from the higher rank. In this nursing school, also, for students of higher ability level, the rate of leaving for those of lower social class was (3 of 14) 21% and for those of higher social class (1 of 7) 14%. Thus, the effect of social class on the student's not completing the program is greater for the low-ability student than for others.

Considering all those who left as the Outs, and all who remained as the Ins, with regard to several questions asked of them at the time they entered school, there was a tendency for Ins to have first considered entering nursing and to have made their final decision at an earlier age than those who left. (Chi-square tests did not reach statistical significance.) To the extent that these choices reflected a commitment to nursing, it may be said that those who reported making an early commitment were more likely to complete the program.

Several characteristics related to academic interest differentiated the two groups. When asked about their plans for further education after nursing school, more Ins (65%) said they planned to seek at least a B.S. degree than did Outs (48%). The Ins (82%) were also more likely to have been in an academic rather than a commercial or general course program in high school than Outs (54%). (This difference was significant at .05 level using Chi-square.) Consistent with this is the fact that 13% of the Ins either considered or had gone to college at least up to the point of taking the entrance exams, in contrast to one girl, or 4%, of the Outs. Similarly, when classified according to alternative occupational careers they had considered, the Ins (45% vs. 22%) were more likely to have considered teaching, whereas the Outs had more frequently considered becoming airline stewardesses (26% vs. 5%). There were no differences on such other occupations as other professions or clerical and secretarial work.

Differences in academic interest and ability are reflected in the distribution of students according to ability level. Some 44% of the Outs were in the lower ability level in contrast to 21% of the Ins. Performance in nursing school, as early as the first quarter, followed the same pattern with up to 65% of the Outs obtaining grades of D or F in one subject, compared with 25% of the Ins. However, both groups had indicated at the time of entry that they expected that their studies would be the most difficult part of nursing school (59% and 54% for the Outs and Ins respectively). Thus, expectation of difficulty is not unequivocally related to actually experiencing academic difficulty.

The social background of the students showed that Ins tended to come from somewhat higher socioeconomic levels than Outs, as measured by father's education and occupation. When each of these was considered separately, the fathers of the Ins more frequently were professional, managerial, clerical and sales persons (48% vs. 30%), and the fathers of Outs were more frequently foremen, operatives and skilled workers (56% vs. 28%). With regard to education, 26% of the fathers of Ins had gone to or completed college in contrast to 8% of the fathers of Outs. More striking is the fact that the mothers of Ins were more likely to have spent some time in college (25%), in contrast to *none* of the mothers of girls who left nursing school.

The mother's occupation, for all instances in which the mother had worked, showed some trend in the direction of mothers of Ins having worked as nurses (3 cases), or medical assistants (3 cases), or having been in professional or managerial kinds of occupations including nursing (17% vs. 4%).

Other background characteristics which were examined but which showed no differences between the two groups were the girl's age, religion, family size, size of home town, size of graduating class and whether the girl had ever lived away from home.

With regard to their expectations for nursing and school, there were no differences between the two groups on questions such as what they expected to like most or like least, whether they expected to work as nurses and to marry, what specialty they might prefer to enter, and how they perceived job opportunities in nursing.

Teal and Fabrizio[10] asked students whether they would choose nursing again. Twenty-eight per cent of all students, including degree and diploma programs, stated that they would not choose nursing if they had it to do over again. Of those who were still in school in the diploma program, 92% said they would. Throughout all programs, academic dropouts were more willing to choose nursing than non-academic dropouts. They comment, and we can concur, that "it is unfortunate that the ones who have trouble academically are the same ones who appear to desire nursing so strongly."

The sum total of these efforts to determine what factors are related to eventual completion or leaving school is mixed. No single factor, other than intellective kinds of variables, showed any strong relationship which might be used in a predictive fashion. Furthermore, even intellective predictors were not consistent in their results or stable in terms of showing the same relationship for first- and second-year dropouts. Clearly, neither a single variable nor a combination of several variables was sufficient to predict to success in the program. Social class and ability level both appear to be important, but it is only the combination of low ability and low social class, that predicts to failure. More of the successful students have academic interests, have mothers and fathers with higher education, and come from generally higher social class levels than do the dropouts. These variables may be of some value in predicting success or failure but the numerous exceptions mean that some girls still manage, despite what might appear to be handicaps, to complete the program.

This analysis seemed to us to show that predictor variables which focused solely on the characteristics of individual students offered little indication of how the student was responding to the school situation and whether she could be helped to remain in school. The student is involved in a complex interactional process, and individual social and personality characteristics offer some clues to understanding this process. However, in order to determine

---

[10] Teal and Fabrizio, *op. cit.*, p. 20.

what the school could do to assist students to complete requirements (without necessarily lowering standards) an intensive analysis of individual cases was undertaken.

On the basis of intellective predictor studies, one might be inclined to conclude that merely selecting students with higher grade point averages in high school would reduce the number of dropouts. We have found, however, that dropping out in the second year shows little relation to intellective predictors. And, more significantly, higher social class position seems to compensate in some unknown way for lower ability levels. Thus, setting higher standards based on intellective criteria for admission to nursing school would exclude some students who otherwise would have little difficulty completing school. Whether these students go on to practice nursing after graduating from nursing school, and how competently they practice, is something that remains to be seen. In this study, we will deal only with completion of school as the outcome criterion since this is a necessary prerequisite to subsequent entry into practice.

OFFICIAL "REASONS" FOR DROPOUTS

In the search for institutional factors involved in producing dropouts, we turned first to an examination of the school's system of classifying dropouts.

A set of categories, used in official reports by the National League for Nursing (NLN), was used by the school to classify the reasons why girls left the school. Although it could be assumed that any institution's classification system could be used in a fashion that would protect it from blame, conceal its least desirable characteristics, and protect its students' reputations, we felt that an examination of the actual cases that were classified in each category would reveal the meaning of that category *as it was used* by the school and also how students were perceived by the school. We knew that we would have to be careful not to interpret the official reasons as the real or only reasons.

In order to provide some evidence that there were different viewpoints, the dropouts themselves were interviewed and asked their reasons for having left school. These reasons and the school's official reasons were tabulated against each other, using the same NLN list, to determine what discrepancies existed. The discrepancies could then be examined to discover why there might be a "distortion" of reasons in the official record. Follow-up interviews were conducted in 1965, some one to two years after these girls had left school. Thus it was also possible to learn of their activities since leaving school, including work, schooling, and marriage.

Table 4 presents a cross-tabulation of data obtained in our study and shows how the school's officially recorded reasons compared with the girl's own story. The categories "marriage" and "dislike of nursing" showed only one instance of disagreement between reasons given by the school and the girl, whereas there was disagreement on all cases listed by the school as "personal" and on a

Table 4. Comparison of School's Recorded Reasons for Dropouts with Students' Reasons

| Official School Record | Girl's Reason | | | | |
	Failure	Marriage	Dislike	Personal and Financial[a]	N
Failure	8	0	3	1	12
Marriage	0	8	0	0	8
Dislike	0	0	7	0	7
Personal and Financial[a]	0	1	2	0	3
N	8	9	12	1	30

[a]For purposes of discussion and analysis, since there were so few cases in the "personal" and "financial" categories, these are subsequently included under the classification of "dislike of nursing." This seems justifiable in light of the fact that the faculty members, describing these instances, reported that the element of dislike was certainly present and two of the three girls interviewed stated that they disliked nursing.

third of the cases listed as "failure" with the latter being viewed by the girl as a dislike of nursing rather than academic failure. One clear finding was that more students were willing to admit to a dislike of nursing than the school was willing to record.[11]

[11] The discrepancy between the student's own reason as given on a mail questionnaire and that reported by the school administration or as found in the school's file was found to be approximately 66% by Teal and Fabrizio, *op. cit.* In this study the rate is only 24%.

Teal and Fabrizio[12] had also investigated the differences between the reasons given by the student for leaving and the official reasons listed by the school. Originally they planned to classify dropouts into three categories: voluntary resignations for personal reasons; involuntary resignations for reasons other than academic failure; and dismissal for academic failure. The first problem they encountered was determining whether the student had left voluntarily. The classification of reasons for leaving used by the school was discovered to be affected by considerations that varied from one school to another so that even "resignation" could be voluntary or requested. The final officially recorded reason often offered no clue to the variety of precipitating factors and to the complex process of withdrawal from school.

In pursuing the effort to classify dropouts, Teal and Fabrizio made the implicit assumption that there is one reason, in fact, they refer to a "primary" reason, which can account for a student's leaving. Other factors become secondary. At the same time they note that it is impossible to determine which reason is the "straw that breaks the camel's back." Despite these difficulties, they proceed to substitute a new set of reasons consisting of some 48 statements, for the old, based on the quoted statements of students who were asked why they had left school. The results of their study are helpful in revealing facets of the process which had not been given explicit attention before, but they are still misleading in that the search for single causes obscures the complexity of the phenomenon being studied. Their approach only substitutes one set of reasons for another. It does not necessarily come any closer to understanding the process of withdrawal from school as a complex sequence of activities involving many steps and many persons. The student's own characteristics, what she is at the time she enters and what she is becoming, also enter into this process in some manner.

By examining each of the official categories and the individual cases within these, we want to show the variety of circumstances that lead to a girl's leaving. No category is revealed to be unitary in the sense of containing cases for which the name of the category could be said to represent "the" reason for leaving. This examination will lead us into the construction of new categories based on multiple factors. Anticipating the step we took after this analysis, we can

---

[12] Teal and Fabrizio, *op. cit.,* p. 13.

say that the final classification we arrived at is not taken to mean that the label assigned to the category is the reason for leaving. The label instead refers to a constellation of factors which were interrelated in such a special way that, operating together, they produced the end result, "dropping out," but the process leading to this result was different from the process involved in each of the other types. But before presenting our system for classifying dropouts, we will show in some detail the variety of types classified under each of the official NLN categories. The deficiencies of this classification system should then become apparent.

FAILURE

There appeared to be at least four kinds of cases within the failure category alone:

1) The first included those girls who would have liked to remain in school, but who indeed could not "make the grade"; that is, girls who had low ability and were not able to perform at a level acceptable to the institution.

2) A second kind included those who also did not do passable work, chiefly because of poor study habits or failure to apply themselves.

3) A third kind included those who failed academically but who also disliked nursing to the extent that they found it difficult to maintain an interest in keeping their grades up. It seems important to point out here that in a case where failure and dislike occurred, failure as a reason for leaving was always given priority in the official school record. Perhaps this was because, from the institution's point of view, it was much more acceptable that a girl leave because of her inability to measure up to the school's standards than because she did not like the institution or the prospect of a nursing career. There is no question that dislike of any task contributes to a reduction of efforts to succeed, yet the present classification system does not take into account the fact that a student may dislike some aspect of the school experience and then, because of her general dissatisfaction, fail in her course work.

4) The fourth kind included those who failed academically, but who also found themselves entangled in other serious problems at home or at school, such as non-acceptance by the rest of their classmates. Such cases could also be classified as failure in the school

record, yet it is interesting to note that of the four girls so classified, three did not tell the interviewer that they failed their course work, but rather attributed their leaving to such things as living away from home, having problems with the director of nursing, and illness in the family.

Of course, there is some justification for this category in that all who were termed failures actually did fall below a certain standard in either classroom or clinical performance or both; i.e., they did have failing averages in a course or courses. However, failure is generally attributed to the student's inability to meet standards and does not consider that a variety of prior events, not just low ability, may lead to or produce failure.

Even though educators and laymen alike classify students according to "flunk out" or "pass" criteria, closer examination of the classification system reveals that a variety of cases are classifiable under the same heading only by stretching the boundaries of the category, selecting certain facts as more significant than others, or reinterpreting the meaning of certain events that have already occurred so that they "fit" the categories available for classification. This process is one in which the pre-existence of a set of categories determines the reality of events since a case can be classified in one and only one category. The meaning of the category is stated in advance and, therefore, a case classified in that category is interpreted according to what the category "means." This labeling process is not, in this instance, as significant for the subsequent life of the individual as it is for persons who are labeled as "criminal" or "mentally ill," since it is not a public label which easily becomes known to others. However, it is of considerable significance for the individual's record in school and for any subsequent re-entry or transfer. It is also important for the individual's self-image in that whatever stigmatic connotations exist can be felt by the individual and can affect her subsequent interactions with others. To be classified as a dropout is somewhat stigmatic in our society, whereas to leave nursing in order to marry is less so. If one knows this, events can sometimes be arranged so that less stigmatic and less ego-damaging reasons may be offered as the reasons for students leaving before completing the program.

MARRIAGE

Some of these points can be illustrated by examining the category "marriage" as a reason for leaving school. Marriage is one of the main reasons for leaving given in official school records. Girls who have enrolled in nursing school after completing their high-school education have, at this point, given priority to some type of further education and have, in a sense, postponed marriage. What is interesting is that so few left this school to marry. As can be noted in Table 4, eight cases were listed as leaving for this reason. The school's reports were corroborated by the girls, although both from the girl's point of view and the school's, there appeared to be several complicating factors which official records simply did not include. Marriage, as a category, consisted of four sub-categories:

1) The first sub-category included girls who preferred marriage to continuing in nursing school and who were forced to make a choice, since it was the school's policy not to allow students to remain in school while married, except for those who married during the last five months of the senior year. (This rule was subsequently changed to allow students to marry at any time provided the school was properly notified.) Some of those who married may have preferred immediate marriage to delaying marriage or to completing school. For example, one instructor said of a girl obviously in this position, "She liked nursing but decided that she would rather be married and raise a family than to continue her education and become a nurse."

2) A second sub-category includes those girls who disliked nursing and who defined marriage in their own minds as an "out," that is, an acceptable way of extricating themselves from the unpleasant and problematic school atmosphere. The circumstances of one girl's marriage point up the fact that marriage seemed to be an answer to her unhappy situation at school. She was doing poorly in course work, had difficulty getting along with her roommate and was ostracized by other class members. When her boyfriend, who was living out-of-town, called her and asked her to marry him, she packed her bags and without any further plans or notification, left school within an hour.

There is, of course, the possibility that the real reason for her marrying was pre-marital pregnancy. Since out-of-wedlock pregnancy would be an embarrassing circumstance for the girl, she would have been disposed to report, in the event of early self-discovery, only that she was leaving school to marry. The school may then have recorded this as the reason for leaving. In some cases where this had occurred, the faculty either had no reason to believe the girl left because she was pregnant or else did not probe more deeply into the question. It would also have been disadvantageous for the school to reveal that they had accepted some girls who showed questionable moral behavior, or that students had misbehaved during their training period.

If school personnel were aware of the fact that a girl was pregnant and either secretly married or planning to be married shortly, the record may have stated "married and pregnant" as the reason for leaving. There were instances when the faculty "covered" for the student by omitting any indication that she was pregnant when she left. Neither the student's nor the school's record was marred when the statement of her pregnancy was omitted. In general, faculty members seemed very unwilling to discuss these instances when the researchers suspected or inferred that the girl may have been pregnant.

3) The third sub-category subsumed under the heading "marriage" included girls who discovered they were pregnant and who either married or announced that they would marry. These girls could present marriage as an acceptable reason for leaving. For example, one girl was described by the faculty as leaving "in order to get married; she was sorry to go, but since hospital policy would not permit her to remain and be married, she chose the latter." This girl, we later learned, was pregnant before marrying but there is no indication from interviews with the faculty or from official records that this was known.

4) The fourth sub-category represents a logical extension of the list. It includes those girls who were pregnant and the school became aware of their circumstances. They were then reported as leaving for reasons of "marriage and pregnancy." It seems that the girls in this position, just as in the case described above, did not necessarily wish to leave nursing school, but had to in light of school policy. One of these dropouts reported to the interviewer about six months after leaving that "if I hadn't become pregnant, I would have kept my marriage a secret and finished nursing school; the school made me leave since being married and pregnant while still in school was against school policy.'"

Thus, marriage, as a category, included several variations. Some students used marriage as a socially acceptable reason for leaving the school so they would not have to admit a dislike for nursing, whereas for others school policy dictated the expulsion or resignation of a student who otherwise would have preferred to stay. It is apparent that the student who knew the school's policy could expel herself by marrying. Wanting to stay but getting married and then having to leave because the rules require it is different from wanting to leave and then getting married in order to make a graceful exit. The former included instances in which the student wanted to and would have completed the program if it were possible to do so; whereas the latter refers to instances in which the student wanted to and perhaps would have left prior to completing the program in any case, but marriage became the ostensive reason for leaving. The former can include those cases in which pregnancy occurred prior to marriage. Eventually, if marriage did not occur, the student would have been asked to leave. Secret marriage, followed by pregnancy, followed by discovery (of either) has the same consequence and may be said to represent the same pattern, i.e., a change in one's status (from non-pregnant to pregnant, or from unmarried to married) which, when discovered, leads to similar treatment. It is also possible that a secret marriage may be known to school authorities and because the girl is outstanding, the rule is not enforced. In our study no cases were found in which this could be said to have happened.

DISLIKE OF NURSING

A number of girls left because they disliked nursing, or were so reported on official records. Within this category, variations that were found included the following:

1) Some girls realized that nursing was not to their liking once they had been introduced to it. They apparently did not know in advance what it would be like. As one girl stated, "I wasn't cut out to be a nurse—I sensed it inside."

When subjected to actual nursing experience, several students found that they were not capable, "couldn't take it," or didn't like dealing with patients. One student described her clinical experiences in the following way: "I left nursing because it made me too nervous when I was on the floor. I enjoyed the classroom and my grades were fine. But in the actual performance of the treatments, I was too afraid I would hurt someone or endanger patients' lives. I could never relax when in the hospital." In these instances, it was not academic performance that was the problem, but rather nursing practice.

2) There were also some girls who admitted, and possibly others who did not admit to the interviewer or to the faculty, that their dislike stemmed from a dislike of nursing *school*, or of this particular school, rather than of the field of nursing. One girl, for example, reported that she told the faculty that the patients depressed her, but the real reason was that:

> I was just fed up with nurses training. A little bit of everything made me fed up. Part of it was the patient problems; you'd work on it all night and the instructor would always find some-thing wrong with it. I like to do good . . . in high school when you do bad, the teachers don't ridicule you but they do in nurses training. They always talk to you like you hadn't studied and didn't know what you were talking about. They picked on you—they did the other girls too but I was sensitive to it.

However, this girl was not considered a good nurse by the faculty because of her desire to keep her distance from patients and her resentment of patient demands. In such cases, it would be difficult for the student to say, in an exit interview with school officials, that it was the instructors or school routine or dormitory living that she disliked. We would expect that if these were the important reasons they would be disguised under some other heading, conceivably even academic failure or marriage.

3) A last sub-category under dislike of nursing is the dislike of being away from home. This could happen regardless of whether the student was in nursing school or some other kind of school. It accounted for only one girl's leaving. This particular student was very homesick; according to the faculty, "She was an only child and went home every weekend." The girl herself said that "living in a city in a two-by-four room got on my nerves."

An examination of the cases grouped under each of the official headings shows that a variety of "types" are included under the same heading and that no category can be said to represent a dis-tinctive constellation of factors that may be used to describe the individual's reason for leaving. Furthermore, there was occasional disagreement between the student's and the school's stated reasons for leaving even when the same set of named reasons was used. This discrepancy may be inevitable since two perspectives were involved.

One other fact about these official reasons should be noted. As they are used and defined, the burden of blame is placed upon the student. It is *she* who fails. Failing is a process in which the student, lacking ability, interest, application or some combination of these three, does not succeed in actively winning the valued grade. On the other hand, there is no category in which the school can be judged as having failed to meet the student's expectations, interests or needs. The school cannot fail; only the student can.

Just as failure is the student's failure, dislike of nursing is a characteristic of the individual; getting married is something the student does either because it is more attractive than nursing or because she has to; personal reasons, financial reasons and health are all obviously the student's problems.

Suppose we were to look at the situation from a different perspective and ask how some of these categories might be labeled from the student's point of view. The counterpart of dislike of nursing would be dislike on the part of the school (i.e., on the part of the faculty, administrators and staff) for the student. Failure would include such things as the school's failure to screen students carefully or to help them overcome "reality shock," or to motivate them sufficiently so that they would persevere. Financial reasons would be seen as a lack or unwillingness of the school to provide assistance to pay for the girl's education. Marriage would be viewed as institutional inflexibility in not allowing students to marry while in school or to continue their education despite pregnancy. In other cases, this inflexibility would be represented by the acceptance of societal mores which do not sanction pregnancy out-of-wedlock or allow abortion, or, prior to this, provide sex education and information concerning birth control. New categories might have to be devised to include restrictive norms which require expulsion or withdrawal when violated. In this latter instance, we have in mind especially those rules that are developed for purposes of keeping order and discipline in the dormitory and for assuring what the institution views as the proper moral conduct of resident students. Such norms have little to do with role socialization but develop out of institutional needs and eventually are defined as relevant for the proper training of the student nurse. Generally, it is the dignity, prestige, or reputation of the school that is alleged to be at stake if students do not conform.

Thus, although the above picture is overdrawn, it is possible to argue that the school is at fault for every case in which a student leaves before completing training. This exaggerated view would be unfair to the school, just as the existing classification system is unfair to the student. A combination of individual and institutional factors in a model which makes meaningful the interactive effects of the two is to be preferred.

If such a combination could be developed, it is likely that it would make sense out of the apparent conflict between reasons for dropping out that are given by the school and those mentioned by the student. It could, hopefully, yield a set of categories that would be theoretically as well as empirically meaningful insofar as it would explain why students leave school. Instead of relying on a single factor explanation, as is the case in the one-word category system presently in use by the National League for Nursing, it could yield a multi-factor system which would come closer to describing the reality of the complex process that is, in fact, involved in a student's leaving school. A model of such a system, using illustrative cases selected from data obtained in our study, is presented below.

MODEL OF A MULTI-FACTOR SYSTEM FOR CLASSIFYING DROPOUTS

What combinations of factors should be included in the model? Our selection was guided in the present instance by what we already knew and we present our analysis not to test some explanatory hypothesis but rather as an effort to make sense out of a multitude of facts.

From the student's perspective, the following factors appear to be important: the degree of interest and motivation for becoming a nurse and the sustaining of such interest and motivation; the perception of the school as providing a desired and understandable sequence of events for the achievement of this goal; the availability of financial support; the presence of or development of friendships with peers; the absence of competing alternatives such as pressures from family, fiancé (or husband) to leave school; and the ability to adjust to the demands of the institution including academic, social and clinical demands.

From the school's perspective, important factors are: the level of the student's intellective ability as measured by entrance examinations or pre-entrance performance criteria (e.g., high-school grades) ; the perceived motivation and suitability (including personality characteristics) for becoming a nurse; the student's performance while in school; and her responses to institutional rules and regulations.

Examining individual cases in terms of these several characteristics, we finally arrived at a typology of five categories. Cases classified under each category seemed to have many characteristics in common. The relation of these categories to the official reasons for leaving, previously discussed, will be noted in passing but, at this point, we can anticipate our findings by saying that there is no direct relation between the two sets of categories. Table 5 presents the names of the categories and a tabulation of the frequency of cases within each. A detailed description of each category, including case history material, follows.

Table 5. Number and Percentage of Dropouts by Category

Category		N	%
I	Academic failure	4	13.3
II	Unsuitable for nursing: forced out	4	13.3
III	Unsuitable for nursing: emotional problems	5	16.6
IV	Dislike of nursing: self-realization (small-town girls = 2)	9	30.0
V	Institutional inflexibility: loss to nursing	7	23.3
	Unclassifiable	1	3.3
		30	99.8

As each type is presented with illustrative cases, it should become clear that our conception of dropouts does not seek to pin blame or find scapegoats. Both the student and the school are responsible, or perhaps we should say involved in the complex process that results in the girl's leaving school. We feel that the types described show more clearly the mutual inter-dependence of the two as well as reveal possible remedies or solutions. This conceptualization provides a better handle for attacking the problem of dropouts because it reveals the manner and extent to which each of the parties is involved in the process. A discussion of the implications of this classification for reducing dropouts is reserved for the conclusion of this chapter.

I: ACADEMIC FAILURE

The first group consisted of students who could be called true academic failures. For all girls so classified the official reason for their leaving was also given as failure. However, not all who were *officially* classified as failures fell into this category. All were in the lowest ability category, received below-average grades in the first quarter of the freshman year and left school because they had received a below-passing grade in one or more subjects. Some left during the first year and some at the very beginning of the second year. None was the target of any strong dislike or active rejection by peers. All were interested in becoming nurses and, even after flunking out of school, sought jobs in which they might work as nurses' aides or doctors' assistants, or in a medical setting. Several sought to re-enter nursing school. Because they were regarded as being deficient in academic ability but not in their desire to become nurses, some were re-admitted to the same school if judged as having a chance of making it on a second try, and some entered other schools regarded as being less difficult than this one. Their compensating feature would be the strength of their desire and motivation. These dropouts may be characterized as academic failures, purely and simply, or as not having "what it takes" to pass the formal academic requirements. However, such judgments should not be unqualified because some dropouts listed in this category might be able to pass the course work if given a second chance.

In one sense, these girls should probably not have been admitted to the school since they were low on the various intellective criteria used by the school in selecting students, i.e., high-school rank, scores on the Nursing Admissions Test and Otis IQ. However, some others who also scored low on these criteria left school for a variety of reasons other than academic failure, so it cannot be said that failure is "purely and simply" related to intellective ability.

In the following case descriptions, some details have been changed to protect the anonymity of the student.

Dropout No. 1: She Had to Leave Because She Failed

This girl was in the lowest ability group. She failed the chemistry course in the second quarter. The official reason for her leaving was "failure." Faculty members who were interviewed agreed that this was the only reason she left. She had been failing and was put on probation at the end of the first quarter; by the end of the third quarter, she was still failing in one or more courses. She didn't seem to know how to study. The faculty felt she could have become a nurse if she could have passed her academic courses.

She first found a job in the rehabilitation unit in another hospital and worked for eight months. Then she entered another nursing school but, after a year, was asked to leave because of a personality conflict with one instructor. The day after she left the instructor was fired. Her grades there were all A's and B's.

She left her job to go back to nursing school because "she always wanted to be a nurse" and could see that "you don't make enough money and there is no chance for advancement unless you are an R.N."

After she left the second school, she became a doctor's assistant filling in for someone else who was on vacation; then she became a "nurses' assistant" in a hospital but this boiled down to being a nurses' aide. "I had expected to be able to do more, but I only made beds, passed trays and visited with patients. I had been taught to do more complex things in nurses' training." She also didn't like being a nurses' aide because she had so little responsibility. "I like a job where you have a little responsibility and where there's some challenge." She then went into private duty nursing for four months until her patient could no longer afford to pay her. The patient's physician then hired her as a nurse in his office. This job is one that she thoroughly enjoys and it seems to be a satisfactory solution to her desire to be a nurse despite not having completed nursing school.

Since leaving nursing school, she has considered going to college to become a physical therapist since she especially enjoyed this kind of work. In the meantime, however, she has married and it would not be financially possible for both herself and her husband, who is still in school, to be in college at the same time. Prior to marrying, she took some courses in the evening program at a local college but was not pursuing a degree.

She received the average number of positive sociometric choices from her peers and no negative choices.

As this case illustrates, little else mattered other than low performance in academic courses. The student's motivation and interest were high as evidenced by her subsequent re-entry into nursing school and her job history. If she had had the manifest ability, that is, not only the capacity to perform but the demonstrated performance, she undoubtedly would have made it through school on the criterion of clinical performance.

These girls were not the most popular and highly chosen students, but neither were they disliked by their peers, i.e., they were not chosen on negative sociometric criteria. They were not maladjusted nor did they show signs of personality disturbance. They represent the group for whom intellective criteria should be able to predict. As noted, they were in the lowest ability group and among the lowest of all members of the class on intellective predictors. They can best be classified as motivated, suitable, but lacking in ability.

II: UNSUITABLE FOR NURSING: FORCED OUT

All of these dropouts were judged to be unsuitable for nursing by virtue of personality, attitude or other characteristics which led the faculty to say they were "glad she left." If the girl did not leave of her own accord, it can be safely predicted that she would have been asked to leave eventually. For these girls, failure in courses represents an active weeding out of those judged unsuitable for nursing. Sometimes one point below passing in one course may be used as a providential opportunity for asking the girl to leave school. Failure, in such a case, is not to be interpreted as *her* failure, but rather that the *school* failed (forced) her out.

Although all professed an interest in still becoming nurses, only one (who had been an L.P.N. before entering) worked or sought work in medical settings after leaving school. All left within the first year. All received the lowest ratings by the faculty on suitability for nursing and, in two of the four cases, were named by over 60% of their peers as the person they "liked least" on the sociometric criteria.

These were students of whom the faculty said: "She failed, thank goodness;" "We were glad when she left . . . if she hadn't married, she may have failed . . . she may have been asked to leave, depending on how she did." Of one who left because of a stated dislike for nursing and for her instructors, they said, "We weren't sorry to see her go. We were delighted when she said she wanted to leave;" and of one who was asked to leave because of a low grade in one course, "She represented almost every possible influence for the bad . . . she was smart enough if she had used her ability, but she was not a good nurse at all."

In short, there was relief rather than concern over these girls' leaving. They could perhaps be classified as the "undesirable ones" that the school would try to force out if at all possible. If they had "made the grade" they would have been the ones that would have been thought of later as casting a bad reflection on the school.

A variety of cases are included under this heading. The official reasons for these girls' leaving are also varied, e.g., failure, dislike of nursing, and marriage are all found under this heading. The common theme, their perceived unsuitability for nursing, can be found in the following descriptions.

Dropout No. 2: She Failed, Thank Goodness

The school officials say this girl "failed, thank goodness." "She had a limited background . . . even though her pre-entrance tests looked adequate. We knew she was limited." Another says, "We had an awful lot of trouble with her not only on her grades, but also on the ward and in the dormitory where she created trouble."

After she left, she went to work as a typist for a year, then left for a better paying job as a secretary. She married and then had a child. At the time she was interviewed, she said she was not working, "just sitting around the house doing housework and going out of my mind." She was looking for a job and planned to return to work soon.

She did not consider entering nursing school again . . . "if I couldn't make it in one school I couldn't make it in another and besides I didn't care that much for it." She had entered nursing not expecting it to be quite so hard. "I expected to have a good time."

Her experiences with faculty and staff were unpleasant and undoubtedly she was aware that she was not well liked. The feeling was mutual. "My supervisor was a witch. I didn't care for her at all. I thought that nurses were supposed to be devoted people and she was the most undevoted woman."

She would not consider any other kind of school, either. "I just wanted to work. I didn't have the money to go to school and there just wasn't anything I really wanted to study." With reference to studies, she commented that one thing she didn't like about nursing school was that "there was so much research to do outside of classes and I hate libraries."

Dropout No. 3: She Was Fed Up with Nurse's Training

The official reason for this girl's leaving was dislike of nursing. The faculty said of her, "This was a funny kid. She was not good, but about average. She was very strange in her relationships with patients. She seemed to prefer to be distant from patients."

"We were delighted when she came and said she wanted to leave because we didn't have much to put our finger on." In other words, it was felt that she was not suitable but there was little that could be offered in the way of reasons for requesting her to leave. She was not failing in her course work.

The girl herself says that she was "just fed up with nurse's training." She told the interviewer that she was depressed but that that wasn't the real reason; part of her dislike was the "patient problems . . . you'd work on them all night but the instructor would find something wrong . . . the teachers ridiculed you . . . they picked on you . . . I was sensitive to it . . . I like to do good and I like people to tell me I do good."

Corroborating the faculty's impression, however, about her having some peculiar attitudes is the following statement that the girl herself made in response to questions asking her whether she was working now that she was out of school and whether she ever did any volunteer work. In response to the question concerning working, she said that she was now a keypunch operator in an office. She expected to stay there "about another two years, and if I'm not making the amount of money I should or don't like the people, I'll probably look for another job. I like the people now, they put up with a lot of stuff that other companies wouldn't . . . like talkin' and goofing off." With regard to volunteer work, she says, "I don't do nothin'. Ever since I was in nurse's training, I don't do anything for anybody unless they ask me and I have to, or I really like them. I don't like worrying for nothing. I would for my friends if they were sick. I'd do their laundry or something like that, but as far as volunteering for other people, I don't think they appreciate it."

One faculty member commented that her attitude "was not particularly good. I'm *not* sorry to see her go." When asked why, she said, "mostly because of her personality. She got angry with patients. She did not like to be asked to do things for patients. She felt that if she gave in to the patients, she would be walked on by them." Thus the faculty members' description is almost the same as the one that the girl gives of herself, i.e., that she does not like to do things for other people.

She was not in the lowest ability group and it is likely that she would have passed her courses. She did not receive many choices on positive sociometric criteria and did receive somewhat more than the median number of least liked choices.

Dropout No. 4: She Was Older, Experienced and a Bad Influence

This girl had worked as a licensed practical nurse before entering the school. She was somewhat older than the other girls. Her past experience and her knowledge of hospital procedures led to her receiving many choices as a preferred teammate on the sociometric test. However, the faculty felt that she was a bad influence on the other girls in that she did not prepare for clinical duty but tried to get by on the basis of what she knew from past experience. She did not attempt "to use principles" which were taught in class.

She was asked to leave because of her grades and her poor clinical performance. She received a grade of 74 in one course, one point below passing and this was "used" as the reason for asking her to leave.

Most relevant is the fact that she clashed with the instructors. She reported this herself when she said that among the reasons for her leaving was that she had many arguments with one of her instructors and that they "didn't get along well . . . we just had a personality conflict. She (the instructor) said I was a leader and that I was leading the girls astray. I was older and the girls would come and talk to me."

This was in fact the case and as the faculty put it, she "represented almost every possible influence for the bad."

She was also regarded as being "anti-authority." She sat in the back of the classroom and did not pay attention, according to one of the instructors. She tried to squeak through on the basis of confidence in her ability but she happened to be in the lowest ability group.

She displayed disrespectful and disobedient kinds of behavior which, in the faculty's eyes, were inexcusable. One such incident was when she refused to report to a member of the faculty who wrote her a note asking her to come in. She denied ever having received the note but had been seen tearing it up in front of all the other girls. This was regarded as an open act of defiance of authority and certainly did not sit well with the faculty.

After leaving, she went back to work as an L.P.N. in a hospital. She applied to another school of nursing but was too late, and their class was full; however, she said she was on their list for the following year, and in the future plans to go ahead and become an R.N.

These three girls represent the actively forced out group of students who were judged by the school to be unsuitable for nursing. In most instances, it appeared unlikely that any school would retain them. Academic failure may or may not have been involved but when it was not, it can safely be said that they would have been failed, i.e., forced out, in some way. No characteristics, measured at the time of their entry into school, could be found which might have served as indicators of their unsuitability. Peer rejection is one factor that appears but this measure was made after they were already admitted.

III: UNSUITABLE FOR NURSING: EMOTIONAL PROBLEMS

The dropouts in this category were also forced out of the school, though not as actively as the girls in the preceding category. These girls tended to have some kind of emotional problem which affected their performance and lowered the faculty's estimation of their suitability. When they encountered difficulty either in their courses or in their clinical performance, they were allowed to leave. There is every likelihood that their emotional problems would have become so great or interfered so much with their performance that they would eventually have been forced by the faculty to leave, although they themselves might not have chosen to do so.[13]

---

[13] Teal and Fabrizio, op. cit., p. 10, noted that there were many emotionally oriented reasons for withdrawal from nursing school for both the academic and non-academic dropouts. "Many of these cases could probably have been salvaged had counseling services outside of the instructor and disciplinary chain been available."

Three of the five girls in this category were in the lowest ability group and two were in the highest group. Ability is not a predictor of the kinds of emotional problems these girls had. All were well liked by their peers and received a substantial number of positive sociometric choices. They tended to be rated by the faculty as low or moderately low on suitability for nursing. They left the school in either the first or the second year.

An indication of their lack of awareness of the problems they had had with nursing was the fact that some of these dropouts sought employment in medical settings and eventually left these jobs also. One girl asked to be re-admitted to the school but was refused; eventually she enrolled in a one-year program for laboratory technicians and completed it. The official reason for her leaving was failure, but she indicated that it was the pressure of the school and the move from a small town to the big city that had created her problems.

Another left officially because of "unsatisfactory clinical work" and was listed as a temporary withdrawal. She constantly suffered from an upset stomach. She admitted that she did not like nursing and, after first working as a laboratory technician in another hospital, took a job as a secretary in an office. School officials said of her that she was "firmly" asked to leave. They felt, at the time, that she did not like nursing but did not know how to get out of it. She was reported to have been relieved when asked to leave. Her parents may have been exerting pressure on her to stay because, after she left, her mother called the school to say that she wanted her daughter to return the following year. The girl, however, never asked to be re-admitted and reported that she never considered entering another school.

In such cases, it appeared that the girl herself was not aware of the source of her emotional problems or that they may have been a response to anxiety. Among the symptoms these girls developed which brought them to the attention of doctors were acute anxiety attacks such as crying, or psychosomatic illnesses, including hysterical conversion symptoms. One girl frequently reported a series of one ailment after another but nothing could be found that was organically wrong.

Though some caution should be introduced, the symptoms these girls developed can be interpreted as responses to the emotional stress that they faced and to their inability to admit, usually to themselves as well as to others, that they did not like the school or nursing. An example of the indirect manner in which such problems may be manifested is the case of one girl listed as having failed. She happened to be in the highest ability group. No one would have predicted that she would fail in her course work. She suffered from psychosomatic ailments and, at the time she left, her problems were compounded by the fact that many members of her family were ill and the family was experiencing financial difficulties. She was also distracted, she said, by being "in love."

There seemed little chance that these dropouts would be re-admitted to nursing school because of their emotional health problems, though interestingly enough, in no case was this the official reason given for a student's leaving. Failure to mention emotional problems on the official record is, in our estimation, a way of "covering" for the girl. Rather than stating this on her record, a more acceptable reason such as failure, or the nondescript "personal reasons," is entered on the schools' records.

The following cases illustrate the types of dropouts classified as unsuitable for nursing.

Dropout No. 5: She Left in a Pique and then Was Sorry

This girl left, according to the faculty, "in great disappointment . . . her major difficulty was in the clinical area." She was a student who didn't want it to be said of her that she was "a poor nurse" though she "did not mind being called a poor student."

The faculty did not seem to be aware that an important factor in this girl's leaving was her emotional involvement with a patient. The girl reported, when asked why she left school, "I became emotionally involved with a patient. When I took care of him, no one in the hospital could control him. They tied him to the bed. My instructor assigned him to me and he responded to me. I had no trouble with him. But as soon as I left him, he would regress. I felt emotionally that he couldn't function without me . . . that no one on the nursing staff or the physicians cared enough about him. I lost a lot of sleep and did a lot of worrying about the old man. When I came into training, all my friends were becoming involved with patients, and I warned them not to, but I found myself doing it."

Another important reason that she mentions was that she was "frustrated with the school, mainly with my instructor; I felt she was picking on me because I knew she didn't like me. Because of her I couldn't get back into training. Also, I was frustrated about the attitude of nurses to patients. For example, the R.N.'s would make fun of patients. The L.P.N.'s and the aides would take better care of patients. The attitude of the school to the students was something else. For example, they first said they would help students in any way that they could and talk to you if you wanted to, but this wasn't true. I tried to talk to the instructor and she was sympathetic to me while I was there, but as soon as I walked out of the room, she didn't care. I knew this by the way she treated me. I talked to another about my grades, but she didn't help much. She gave me a book on how to study and that was the extent of it. I was just disappointed about becoming an R.N."

She applied for re-admission approximately one week after leaving. However, the faculty felt that she should not be re-admitted and told her that she should wait a year. The reason for not re-admitting her was that it would set a bad precedent and would be unfair to the other girls; that is, a student who leaves in a pique should not be allowed to apply for re-admission a week later.

After leaving, she worked as a receptionist and bookkeeper in a doctor's office. She later took a job as a file clerk in the records room of a hospital and finally left medical settings to become a bookkeeper in an advertising agency.

When asked about the future, she said that she would like to go back into nursing sometime and perhaps work as a nurses' aide. Significantly, her ambition is to work as a nurses' aide in an "old folks' home."

She said that when she got out of high school she had had no plans to enter nursing school, but her mother had urged her to take the entrance exam. She didn't want to start working right away so she entered nursing school. One thing that did influence her decision was that nurses had helped both her mother and father so much when they were patients in the hospital. She was well liked by her peers and received no negative sociometric choices. About a year after leaving school, she married and continued to work.

Dropout No. 6: She Found Out that Nursing Was Not for Her

This girl left ostensibly because she was failing. She reported that she probably would have stayed if her grades had permitted, even though she didn't care for nursing. The faculty reported that "she wouldn't be a good nurse at all."

The girl herself came to realize that nursing was not for her. She reported, for example, that she was "much better adjusted after I left. I was much happier. I wasn't as nervous and my health improved. I couldn't sleep or eat. I was having terrific headaches and I haven't had any since I left school. I had to go to bed with them, they were so bad."

She did not consider going back to school again, nor did she apply to any other school.

Thus, though not actively forced out, these girls were not helped to overcome their emotional problems, problems which appear to have been situationally specific rather than pervasive personality disturbances. They were either not judged worthy of help or, because of the lack of adequate counseling services, help was not available.

IV: DISLIKE OF NURSING: SELF-REALIZATION

The girls in this group of dropouts discovered that they did not like the nursing school or nursing. This discovery occurred only after entry and some experience in the program. Some left during the first year of school; others during the second. The reasons they mentioned for leaving were varied but generally were the same as the reasons that had been officially recorded—either dislike of nursing or failing in course work.

They were generally not in the lowest ability group though their grades were not among the highest. In fact, most of them had first quarter grade point averages below the median of the class. They tended to be well liked by their peers with a rare exception. They were regarded as suitable for nursing by the faculty and some of them obtained relatively high ratings on this criterion.

When they left school, none of them went into any kind of work that could be regarded as related to nursing or medicine. They took jobs as receptionists, bookkeepers, secretaries, cashiers and stenographers. Their work history reflected the availability of jobs rather than an interest in helping people.

These are not girls about whom the faculty would say, "We were glad she left," but rather they would comment that "she was an excellent student, a nice person, a loss to nursing . . . a delightful kid"; "a good student who simply did not like nursing"; "a lovely girl . . . left because of failure but with another year of experience, she might have done well." Some of these girls were regarded as not among the best prospects for becoming nurses. For example, one was described as not having a "realistic view of nursing" and another as having "a hard cover" or an "attitude that things didn't matter very much."

In short, these girls were not forced out by the school but tended to remove themselves because of the self-realization or implicit awareness that they were not cut out to be nurses. The faculty had hopes for some of them and felt that they might have been able to make the grade, so to speak, but apparently little was done to reach these girls early enough or at the point when they first began to realize that nursing might not be the most satisfactory career for them. It is questionable whether or not they could have been "saved," but in view of the fact that some of these girls were rated high on suitability for nursing, it would appear that there was some chance that they could have been induced to stay in school, or perhaps to return. On the other hand, from the girl's standpoint, the lack of interest in nursing affected her motivation to perform and could conceivably have resulted in her eventual withdrawal from the field.

Included in this group are two girls of whom it could be said that neither school nor nursing itself was the source of their discontent. Both were doing well in their courses, and were in the highest ability group. They received high ratings from the faculty on suitability but left because the total situation of being in the school, away from home and in the city was more than they could handle. These girls both indicated that they "didn't like the city," thus their dislike was not of the school per se, nor of nursing per se, but of the situation of being away from their small-town homes.

At first glance, there seems to be little that the school can do to help such students to adjust. If the major difficulty is that they are in a large, strange city, away from home, parents and family, it is possible that they never would become adjusted to a nursing school located in a city. One could say that they should never have been admitted but, again, there were other girls in this class who came from small towns and who did adjust and learn to like living in the city. If some students can adjust to life away from home and family, it may be possible to assist others to do so.

Some of the girls in this category appear similar to those in category II. One major difference is that all girls listed in this category were aware of the reasons for their problems. They may also have experienced psychosomatic symptoms in response to emotional stress and, though they may not have fully understood the meaning of these symptoms, they were aware of their discomfort in nursing situations and of dissatisfaction with various nursing experiences. The fact that they did not try to re-enter any nursing school or work in nursing or medical settings is an indication that they were more aware of their problems than the girls in the preceding group. Some were considered by the faculty to be potentially good nurses and therefore a loss to nursing. This type of girl would appear to resemble those in category V (real loss). The major distinction, however, is that the dropouts classified here under dislike of nursing did not feel that nursing was something they wanted to do, whereas those in category V were persons about whom both the faculty and the student agreed that the student did want to become a nurse and to complete her training.

Dropout No. 7: She Did Not Enjoy Nursing Activities

This girl left, according to the school's official record, because of a dislike of nursing. She was regarded as an "excellent student, a nice person, and probably a great loss to nursing. She was a delightful kid."

The rating she received concerning her suitability for nursing was above the median.

The student herself stated that she "didn't enjoy any of the things that a nurse does. I made it through the first year because it was mostly book work and we didn't do much work on the floor. When we started working on the floor . . . the hospital isn't the most pleasant place to work . . . there is pressure especially from instructors. I didn't enjoy doing any of the things a nurse does. If it hadn't been for the pressure from the instructors, I would have stayed in, though I still didn't like the clinical work of nursing. The instructors were always standing over you, watching what you were doing, and they never praised you. They were criticizing everything. They left too much up to the girl to do instead of giving instructions in class."

She said that when she had finished high school, her mother strongly encouraged her to become a nurse. She had been debating whether to enter nursing or teaching, and now says, "If I had it to do over again, I would go into teaching." She was well liked by her peers and received no votes on the least-liked criterion. She was in the middle ability category and was not failing in her course work, in fact, had received grades above the median for her first quarter and for the first year. She left a few months after the beginning of the second year.

Her family was quite upset about her leaving, and her father sold her car as punishment. She went to a junior college for one semester to take courses in typing and shorthand in order to prepare herself for finding a job, since she had been unable to find work without these skills. Once acquiring them, she found employment as a secretary.

The next case represents a student who left primarily because of an inability to adjust to living away from home and being in a large city. As she herself stated, it is probably true that if she had gone to a school "closer to home" she would have completed nursing training.

Dropout No. 8: She Wanted to Be a Small-Town Girl

This girl was described on the school's official record as having left for "personal reasons" which were elaborated as "homesickness." She had had no difficulties with grades and was in the higher ability group.

The faculty rated her above the median on suitability for nursing and felt that the reason for leaving was primarily that she missed being home. Another instructor says that the reason that she left was that she "did not like nursing, it was not for her."

The student herself thought that the reason for her leaving was ". . . lived on a farm all my life and loved the country and being in the city in a two-by-four room with cars, noise, etc., got on my nerves. That was the main reason I quit. There were no other reasons; it wasn't my grades or my studies. Had I gone to a school closer to my home I probably would have stayed because I wouldn't have been living in such a large city."

After leaving school, she found work as a clerk and later married. At the time of her interview, she was at home with a child. She planned to devote her time to being a housewife and mother for a while but thought that she might return to a medical setting to work as a nurses' aide sometime, perhaps after the baby was older. She seemed to be fairly well settled as a housewife, and it is unlikely that she would return to pursue any formal training as a nurse. If she does work, it will probably be part-time and for financial reasons.

While in school, she received the average number of positive sociometric choices, and some negative sociometric choices.

This seems to be a girl who could have been helped, had she stayed in school, in spite of her adjustment problems. However, she did not make her problem known to the counselors or the school personnel, so that they might have taken some measures to help her.

In another sub-group within this larger category are two girls who, although they did not explicitly state that they did not care for nursing, showed such lack of interest, motivation and emotional satisfaction that they failed in their course work. They were not among the poorer students and it is quite likely that they could have satisfactorily completed the course. One of these was dropout No. 9.

Dropout No. 9: She Could Not Take a Poor Evaluation

This girl failed one of her courses, was put on probation in the fourth quarter of the first year, and left in the second year. One faculty member said of her, "If she had used all the ability that she had, she might have made a good nurse but she didn't put forth the effort."

The girl reported that the main reason she left was because of her grades. "I had a chance to bring up my grades but I didn't think the effort was worth it. It seemed like the harder I tried, the worse off I got."

A precipitating problem was that she received a negative evaluation from an instructor and this apparently caused her considerable concern. "I didn't think about leaving seriously until I got the bad evaluation. I thought that if one instructor didn't think that I was capable of doing the work, maybe I wasn't capable. I liked being witht patients, I liked to help them and be sympathetic with them, but I just felt that I probably wasn't suited for it. And I didn't like having as many superiors and bosses as I had. Nursing was a big responsibility, too. I'm still not absolutely positive that it was not for me, for I liked to work with the patients. I'm still a little fuzzy as to exactly why I left, but I would never go back in because once you fail at something it's hard to try it again."

Later she added, "For the year and a half that I was in school, I wasn't sure that I wanted to leave and I still wasn't sure when I left, but after I was home and working, I knew I had done the right thing. I just don't think that I really wanted to be a nurse."

The variation within this category revolved around a common theme: a lack of interest in nursing and lack of motivation or desire to become a nurse. This became greater after exposure to nursing school and clinical experiences. Obviously, some interest and motivation were originally present or the girls would never have applied, but rather than being developed and strengthened, interest and motivation diminished. They were "good kids" but somehow judged themselves to be not "cut out" for nursing.

V: INSTITUTIONAL INFLEXIBILITY: REAL LOSS TO NURSING

This last group represents a fairly distinct category of dropouts who can be called a "real loss" to nursing. They are students who left school, not so much out of any choice of their own, but because the rules did not allow them to stay. Specifically, the rule involved was the one pertaining to marriage and pregnancy. Actually, there were two rules. The first rule stated that a student could not marry except in the last five months of her senior year. The second rule, somewhat implicit instead of explicit, stated that a student could not be' pregnant and remain in school. It was possible, however, for a student to be married within the last five months, become pregnant, and complete her education. The pregnancy of five months presumably would not be visible enough to cause any consternation to the school which, as a rule of thumb, allowed a pregnant student nurse to appear in uniform as long as she was "presentable."

Pregnancy occurring outside of marriage was, of course, frowned upon and an unmarried student discovered to be pregnant would automatically be requested to leave.

The girls in category V, particularly those who left in the third year, were regarded as among the best students in the school. There was every expectation, on their part as well as the school's, that they would complete their education. However, they married for one reason or another and then had to leave. In one case, a girl was secretly married before the beginning of her third year and managed to keep this fact concealed for several months, but then became pregnant and had to leave.

These girls were all generally in the highest or middle ability levels, had been obtaining above average grades, had received an above average number of positive sociometric choices, and were rarely chosen as persons who were least liked by their peers.

Their ratings on suitability for nursing, made by the faculty, were among the highest received by any of the girls who left school. They also strongly desired to be nurses. This is evident in their choice of work after leaving school and in the case of one girl who transferred to a school that allowed students to marry. Others worked as nurses' aides, x-ray or laboratory technicians, or secretaries in medical settings. Since some had to leave because of pregnancy, they did not go to work immediately, but planned to work after the baby arrived. Others were already caring for a young infant and planned to return to work at a later time. None were dissatisfied with nursing as a field of work and all would consider entering nursing again.

This combination of characteristics clearly defines this group of girls as lost to nursing because of restrictive rules concerning marriage and pregnancy. It is possible that other rule infractions could have occurred and that a student who was otherwise qualified, motivated and performing adequately would have been asked to leave. In this sense, the category could be more general and include those who leave for reasons other than marriage or pregnancy. It could also refer to losses due to behavior unrelated to the specific demands of the role, provided the student is otherwise doing satisfactory work; for example, violation of dormitory rules or participating in a student demonstration. However, no instances of misconduct, in this sense, were found among these girls.

In this group, then, are the dropouts who undoubtedly would have graduated and become good nurses. The change in the rule which the school finally instituted will prevent some of these losses in the future. The loss amounts to approximately 25% of those who dropped out of school, or approximately 10% of the entering class. It can safely be said, after examining the case histories of these students, that they did not marry in order to escape from nursing, nor did they marry because marriage was perceived as a more attractive alternative to nursing. They married simply as a matter of course, as would be expected of normal young women at this age, and then encountered the restrictive rule which did not allow them to continue in the school.

Many of them stated rather determinedly that they plan to become nurses still. For example, one said, "I'm going to go back to nursing school and be a nurse even though the school I went to before won't take me back. They want me to wait until my youngest child is in school. By that time, I would have forgotten all I knew." Another states, "I always wanted to be a nurse and I still do." And still another, "As soon as I get my R.N., I want to get a B.S. degree so I can teach."

Included among dropouts in this category are the occasional cases of students who become pregnant first, then marry and leave school. The official reason that may go on their records if the school is aware of the pregnancy is "married and pregnant." Some of these are quite involved cases in which considerable covering of the facts is engaged in by both the student and the school. Such cases would be classified in this category only if they represent a loss as evaluated by the faculty, i.e., the feeling that the girl would have been a good nurse and that it was unfortunate that she left. If other factors were of greater importance such cases might be classified in any of the other four categories. Therefore, it is not the simple fact that a rule is violated but the concomitant absence of other distinguishing characteristics that would lead us to classify someone in this category.

The case presented below illustrates the somewhat atypical case of a student who had married secretly and left when her marriage became known. In other respects, she is similar to the other girls in this category.

Dropout No. 10: She Could Not Keep Her Marriage a Secret

This girl was secretly married while in school and undoubtedly would have finished without revealing to the faculty that she was married, but she became pregnant in her third year of school. She went to a junior college and applied for admission to their nursing program, but was told that she should "just think about having the baby." The junior college accepted married students and allowed pregnant women to drop out and come back to finish their education after the baby was born.

There were some financial problems for this student and some question as to whether she would be able to complete her nursing training right away. She thought of working as a practical nurse for a while in order to earn enough money to complete her training. She said she did not expect to continue to work as a practical nurse because she is much more interested in professional nursing and feels that she would not be satisfied with anything else.

She was in the highest ability group and had no difficulty with her course work. "I thought it was easier than I had expected it to be, both academically and clinically," she said of the program. Her grades in her first year were above the median for her class.

She was given the highest possible rating on her suitability for nursing. She was close to the median but below it in terms of number of positive sociometric choices received from her peers. She received no negative choices.

In short, she was a good student, highly regarded, and competent in her clinical performance, but had to leave because she married.

CONCLUSIONS AND IMPLICATIONS

One conclusion we have drawn from this analysis is that the nursing school is not able to cope with the problem of dropouts because the problem is not adequately understood. We have come to this conclusion because it was only after careful analysis and examination of individual cases that we could determine what the variety of dropouts were like and how those who are classified together are similar. The school lacks a conceptualization of types of dropouts for which different treatments would be prescribed. No specification concerning differential treatment for different types has been presented in the research literature. In fact, previous research has usually fostered the view that dropouts are all alike by virtue of the label assigned to them.

In the group we studied there are clearly some girls that this school, or any school, would reject or force to leave. Girls in the academic failure category represent a type that is judged by the school as unable to meet its requirements; those in the unsuitable for nursing category are eliminated for various reasons—particularly general, global evaluations of the student's ability to adjust to the requirements for student and nurse role performance; those classified as leaving for emotional reasons can also be seen as lacking in the characteristics and performances deemed necessary by the school; whereas in the last two categories, dislike of nursing: self-realization, and institutional inflexibility: loss to nursing, there are strong indications that the school can modify some of its practices and thereby assist the student to remain. Nevertheless, there is a choice involved. Assuming that they could in fact prove effective in reducing dropouts, the recommendations suggested here and in Chapter 7 may not be chosen because the institution prefers to maintain screening procedures and evaluation by trial performance under conditions that are as rigorous and as consistent as possible within a particular educational philosophy. This is a matter of choice. The costs of the present system can be seen in some of the cases described above. Changing the present system may, as some would argue, produce a relaxation or lowering of standards. However, our intention in this analysis is not to suggest changes which would reduce standards, but rather to show that there are alternative procedures and institutional arrangements which could operate to reduce the number of dropouts. Implementing such changes without lowering standards would remain a practical problem, to be solved only with considerable effort.

It is clear from the preceding analysis that different approaches are necessary since a variety of categories of dropouts exists. The analysis shows that blame cannot be placed solely on either the individual or the institution. One who attacks the dropout problem must recognize that the phenomenon of dropping out of school is not an individual act but rather that it involves a relationship between an individual and a social system. Relying on better selection procedures or using predictive tests or criteria ignores the fact that once the student is admitted to the school a relationship is begun which involves fitting the individual into an ongoing social system. How is that process carried on? What attention is given to the adjustment of the individual to the system? What degree of flexibility does the system itself possess which will facilitate individual adjustment? How are problems that emerge confronted and resolved? How are such problems defined in the first place and where is the responsibility for their solution placed?

These are all relevant questions for research. The search for predictor variables, measured by examining the individual prior to or at the time of entrance, needs to be supplemented with a more intensive study of the individual and the institution. A moratorium could be declared on the search for single predictor variables and, if this were done, other avenues of investigation would be stimulated. The results of the present investigation show that a multipronged attack on the problem of dropouts is necessary. The delineation of some of the types of dropouts shows that there is considerable variation within this group. Consequently no single approach to the problem can be expected to succeed.

At this point we can go a bit further and try to indicate the implications of these findings for schools of nursing.

First, with regard to screening errors, little room for improvement in terms of selection on intellective criteria appears likely. Rather, the problem is to capitalize on the high motivation of those students with low academic ability or performance ratings in order to help them make the grade. For the students in the academic failure category, counseling to help them overcome blocks to learning and acquiring study skills can be effective. Tutoring in academic subjects by their classmates or more advanced students can be of specific assistance when they are having difficulty with a particular course.

Another type of screening error is represented by the student who drops out because of emotional problems. Interviews by clinicians or nursing faculty trained to look for emotional disturbances that are of direct relevance to nursing role performance would be helpful in discovering those students whose problems are of such magnitude as to make them unsuitable for nursing. This does not mean that all of the dropouts included in category III should have been denied admission. In fact, psychological counseling, on an individual or group basis, might have been instrumental in helping some of these girls to overcome their fears, anxieties, and disabling emotional responses to the stress of the school and clinical situation. Such counseling could allow the determination of the extent to which the emotional response could be overcome. It is possible that some of these students could have been helped sufficiently to complete their studies and counseled into non-hospital nursing situations or specialties within nursing to which they could make an adjustment. An additional implication is that their emotional responses may have been a reaction to specific features of the nursing school experience rather than a representation of a relatively enduring personality disturbance. If so, there is every reason to expect that they could have been helped with some short-term treatment or counseling.

The girls who do not "fit" into a particular school's routine, or who do not meet its standards for performance, could conceivably succeed in other schools. For these girls, some of whom are found in the unsuitable for nursing category, the school could make concessions or adaptations. If the cost of these concessions is too great, then the loss of the student is inevitable. Not all individuals who have the talent and other attributes necessary to become good practicing professionals can be expected to make a perfect adjustment to any school, no matter how it is run. Here the problem is one of matching the individual's characteristics and interests with the social environment of the school. Some persons can adjust more easily to one type of institution than to another. Unfortunately, there is no classification of schools that would enable us to say what kind of person is best suited to meet the demands of a certain type of institution. Perhaps some day it will be possible to make this assessment. Until then, the school will have to bear the losses involved in admitting students who cannot or will not adjust to the school's expectations and demands.

Related to this is the possibility of counseling students to enter other diploma schools or to modify their aspirations and enter training courses for L.P.N.'s or aides. At another end of the continuum, some students should be counseled to enter collegiate programs which presently offer more intellectual and academic challenge. There is also no reason why diploma schools cannot maintain liaison with other schools to facilitate the transfer of students when this seems advisable.

The danger in making a willing concession to bear the cost of losses of students is that the school can rationalize the status quo. "If students can't adjust to us, tough." Alternative institutional arrangements are unlikely to be considered or ever attempted. As was seen in our discussion of category V, the change in one rule—that prohibiting marriage—can reduce the loss of dropouts by almost one-fourth. Here the decision is relatively easy to make, especially since societal norms are increasingly tolerant of pregnancy in the married student or worker. Other re-arrangements, such as allowing students to live outside of dormitories, changing the curriculum of the school to accommodate transfer students or allowing students to repeat courses previously failed, hit at the core of institutional arrangements and are less likely to be changed. Nevertheless, such changes could have an effect on retaining students or, at least, facilitate the making up of credits. At present, the structure of the curriculum is such that it is impossible for the student to repeat a course in a succeeding quarter, so the student who fails must either leave or (rarely) be asked to make up the entire year. This is hardly a curriculum structure that provides adequate opportunity for the individual to recover from a course deficiency. The student should not be subject to an arrangement that allows a failure in one course to determine her career.

Why should a group of students in nursing school be treated as a "class" that enters, follows the same sequence of courses, and leaves at the same time? Most other educational systems do not operate in this way and, consequently, it is possible for their students to re-take a course or make up a failure. Revision of the nursing school curriculum along these lines would allow some students who now have to leave, to stay. Currently, the organization of academic courses, clinical experience and class schedules is based on the traditional assumption that an ordered, cumulative sequence of courses and experiences is the most effective mode of educating nurses. Because the school is a social system, the readjustment of any one part affects the whole, and small changes are not really small. Nursing education can be reorganized in a manner that provides flexibility for meeting the needs of many different individuals uniquely and creatively. The attempt to make students "fit in" can result in their being "forced out."

A full discussion of the implications of these suggestions is reserved for a concluding chapter. At this point, however, we can note that the evidence shows that schools can do much more than they are now doing to assist the student to complete the program. A departure from the position that only an improvement in selection procedures can reduce the dropout rate is greatly needed.

Chapter 4

Images of Nursing

Students' responses to a series of photographs depicting hospital scenes (the Role Projective Test) are analyzed to determine how perceptions changed from freshman to senior year.

In their relationships with patients, freshmen show greater concern (than seniors) with problems and difficulties of nursing practice but have optimistic expectations concerning outcomes. In relatively undefined situations, freshmen see themselves as frightened, nervous and uncertain when performing tasks that have become, for the seniors, normal nursing experiences.

In their relationships with physicians and interns, a pervasive theme of the students' responses was that of a romantic interest and involvement. Also, seniors are less likely than freshmen to describe themselves as valuable contributors to the physician in providing patient care.

The patterns for all students tested show a striking consistency. Youthful idealism and optimism change to realism based on experience and perceptions of nursing as-it-is. The meaning of these findings for the understanding of the socialization process is discussed in this chapter.

The student nurse's perception of her role relationships with significant others, i.e., doctors, nurses, fellow students and patients, forms one basis for her activities in relation to these others. Her perceptions can be expected to change as she progresses through school, acquires experience in dealing with the variety of situations that occur in the hospital, and develops confidence and competence. In this chapter, we examine how these perceptions of role relationships change during the course of the nurse's training and interpret the meaning of these changes.

Intensive studies of medical students by Becker and others[1] have revealed that entering students are characterized by what may be called idealism, but that as they go through the school experience, they develop cynical feelings in specific situations which are directly associated with their medical school experience, although they never lose their original idealism about the *practice* of medicine. Moreover, their expressions of cynicism or idealism vary not only with the objects of these attitudes (e.g., the specific situation or role relationship) but also with the audiences the individuals have in mind when the attitudes are adopted (e.g., other students, instructors or the lay public). Certain aspects of the beginning students' idealism are found to be irrelevant in the school situation and such realistic attitudes as "getting through school" become more salient.

In this view, idealism or cynicism do not represent personality traits or enduring and persistent value orientations, and any characterization of them which ignores their situationally relevant features would be misleading. Other researchers have been less concerned with the situational basis of such expressions as cynicism and idealism, and have implicitly, if not explicitly, been concerned with the significance of such attitudes for high standards of performance. This is reflected in the concern expressed when the senior or graduate does not show the same humanitarian or idealistic outlook that he had when he entered school. Presumably, the school must have had a negative or undesirable effect if such obviously desirable perspectives have been lost. The effect of such attitudes on the individual's performance of his occupational role, it is im-

---

[1] Becker, H. S., Geer, B., Hughes, E., and Strauss, A., *Boys In White,* University of Chicago Press, Chicago, 1961; and Becker, H. S. and Geer, B., The Fate of Idealism in Medical School, *American Sociological Review, 23,* pp. 50–56, 1958.

plied, will be negative; he will not be as interested in or concerned for his patients; he will perhaps become discouraged in his practice and decline in his dedication to high standards of job performance.*

Eron[2] was among those who focused on cynicism and humanitarianism as individual traits or attitudes. He developed measuring instruments which he applied to his studies of medical, law and nursing students. In his first study of medical students, he found that seniors were significantly higher on cynicism scores and that, although the differences between freshman and senior scores on the humanitarian scale were insignificant, the freshmen scored somewhat lower on this scale (contrary to what was expected). In a second study, Eron[3] reported that freshman nurses were about the same as freshmen medical students on cynicism, but senior nurses were less cynical than senior medical students.

On humanitarianism, the freshmen nurses scored higher than freshmen medical students, but as seniors, they both obtained about the same scores. The results when the study of law students were included were not consistent enough to warrant the conclusion that training or educational experiences operated consistently to produce changes in these two attitudes. The nurses tested by Eron[4] included graduate nurses who had completed their education and freshmen and sophomores in collegiate programs. When the nurses were compared among themselves it was found that cynicism scores were significantly lower for the more advanced students, a pattern which is directly opposite to that observed for medical students. For humanitarianism, third-year graduate nurses scored significantly lower than first-year graduates and collegiate freshmen. Brooks,[5]

---

* The notion that individual personality or attitude characteristics are sufficient to sustain such performance overlooks the relevance of social structural sources of support arising from the work setting, the profession and the peer group. Becker and his associates are among the few that have given explicit attention to these sources.

[2] Eron, L. D., Effect of Medical Education on Medical Students' Attitudes, *Journal of Medical Education, 30,* 1955, pp. 559–556.

[3] Eron, L. D., The Effect of Medical Education on Attitudes: A Follow-Up Study, *Journal of Medical Education, 33,* Part II, 1958, pp. 25–33.

[4] Eron, L. D., The Effects of Nursing Education on Attitudes, *Nursing Research, 4,* 1955, pp. 24–27.

[5] Brooks, B. R., Student Attitudes: How They Change, *Nursing World, 134,* 1960, pp. 24–27.

however, using Eron's humanitarianism scale, found that after one academic year, student nurses in the different kinds of nursing education programs did not show significant changes when pre- and post-test scores were compared although the direction of change was consistently toward a lower score on humanitarianism. It is possible that if a longer follow-up period had been used, significant changes would have been observed.

Among the studies of student nurses is one by Meyer[6] in which photographs depicting different preferred interaction situations were utilized. In cross-sectional samples of students in different years in school, Meyer found that one effect of nursing education on attitudes was that the students' preferred nursing situation shifted from Type I, the "ministering angel" who prefers to be with the patient alone, to such other types as "sharing the patient with fellow workers" or "supervising other workers." Entering students in three kinds of schools—collegiate, diploma and associate degree—as well as high-school students in Future Nurse Clubs, all preferred the "ministering angel" situation, with no significant differences appearing between the various groups. The preferences of students in the collegiate program moved away from the "unaided patient care" situation toward one which placed greater emphasis on sharing the patient; those of diploma school and degree program students moved toward a more colleague-oriented and, to some extent, administrative approach. This can be interpreted as a change from the idealistic perception of the nurse as one who derives satisfaction from working closely with the patient, to the realistic perception of the hospital nurse as a member of a coordinated team providing patient care, with a considerable amount of her time being spent administering the activities of members of that team.

In a study reported by McPartland *et al.*,[7] students in different kinds of nursing schools were asked to "describe the kind of person [they thought] would make an ideal nurse." Freshmen and seniors differed in that freshmen conceived of the ideal nurse in nontechnical, personal terms (59%), whereas seniors used technical or

---

[6] Meyer, G. R., *Tenderness and Technique: Nursing Values in Transition,* Los Angeles Institute of Industrial Relations, University of California, 1960.

[7] McPartland, T. S. *et al., Formal Education and the Process of Professionalization: A Study of Student Nurses,* Publication 107, Community Studies, Inc., Kansas City, Missouri, 1957, p. 54.

professional criteria to describe her (57%). When asked to indicate how and in what way their conception of nursing and the nurse had changed while in school, senior respondents indicated a shift from "positively evaluated personal attributes" toward "task-centered descriptions and negatively-toned evaluations." The data are interpreted as showing that:

> . . . direct experience with the work of an occupation results in the revision of idealized conceptions in the direction of the realities of that occupation. . . . Soon after entry into a school of nursing the image of the nurse . . . shifts away from idealization of the nurse toward awareness of the tasks of the nurse or toward negatively toned judgments about some nurses, at least. These shifts may be regarded as shifts toward reality. They are commonly, but not universally, reported by students. . . . Some students retain idealized images and give no attention to the tasks of the nurse (25.8%) and some either retain or acquire negatively toned images of the nurse (24.2%).

In a 3-year follow-up study of students in a collegiate program, Olesen and Davis[8] analyzed the responses to a 19-item check-list of characterizations of nursing and found that there was a decrease in idealism and an increase in realism as the students progressed through the program. Respondents were asked to indicate whether an item corresponded with their picture of nursing and whether it was important to them personally. Some of the items were: dedicated service to humanity; exercise of imagination and insight; meticulousness; close supervision and direction, and job security. One item which showed a decrease in the degree to which it was attributed to nurses was "dedicated service to humanity," a decline which the researchers attributed to a readjustment of romanticized versions of the field, as well as to "reality shock." Although the response to a single item cannot be accepted as definitive, this item showed a decline, though not a significant one, in the *first* year of nursing school.[9]

---

[8] Olesen, V. and Davis, F., Baccalaureate Students' Images of Nursing: A Follow-up Report, *Nursing Research, 15,* 1966, pp. 151–159.

[9] Davis, F. and Olesen, V., Baccalaureate Students' Images of Nursing: A Study of Change, Consensus and Consonance in the First Year, *Nursing Research, 13,* 1964, pp. 8–15.

Willman[10] found that significant changes occurred in the responses of student nurses at three levels in diploma and degree programs. Freshmen's responses reflected their naivete, insecurity, inexperience and self-centered concerns; juniors' responses expressed general discontent and disillusionment with nursing and nursing education in combination with a more realistic conception of nursing; and seniors' responses showed the development of a broader understanding of nursing and of the nurse's' functions and responsibilities.

In general, the results of these studies showed an increase in cynicism or realism as the student moved through school. Studies of medical students and nursing students do not always show the same patterns, however. Aside from the different kinds of nursing schools studied, other factors that may account for the diversity of findings are the lack of good designs which would permit a less equivocal assessment of the effect of the school experience on changes in attitudes (longitudinal studies would be extremely helpful), and the inconsistent use of measuring instruments. Different studies have used different approaches to the measurement of the variables discussed. Rather than arguing for the standardization of tests to measure humanitarianism and cynicism, however, we need to study how these attitudes are manifested in the performance of the incumbent of the role in specific situations.

Other than Becker and his associates, most researchers have not been concerned with the situationally specific aspects of the attitudes studied. Humanitarianism, idealism, or cynicism are regarded as global characteristics, for example, or as orientations which would be expected to have a pervasive effect on a variety of behaviors. As Becker *et al.* have noted:

People ordinarily think of cynicism and idealism as general traits of persons. The cynic so conceived is a man who has no belief in the ultimate worth of what he is doing and no interest in doing good to others; the idealist, a man who thinks his work worthwhile and who wants to help others. According to this view, these attitudes inform every area of a man's thought and activity. It is more likely that these are not general traits but ways of looking at people and situations. Consequently, they

---

[10] Willman, M. D., *Attitudes and Problems of Student Nurses,* Austin, Texas, University of Texas, Ph.D. dissertation, 1961.

vary according to the person or situation one is looking at. A student may be cynical about some things but quite idealistic about others. Those studies in which students' "cynical" attitudes are measured by asking them to agree or disagree with general statements about human nature (such as: "Most people are out for what they can get") obscure this point by not taking account of the specific referents of the attitude. A person's attitude may be cynical or not, depending upon the audience to whom he is interpreting his actions. He may speak cynically to an audience of peers but idealistically to an audience of laymen, or he may do the reverse. We should recognize that cynicism and idealism are not general attributes of the actor, but judgments made by either the actor or someone else about his activity and feelings in certain circumstances. No act or attitude is in itself cynical or idealistic. It depends upon the situation and how one looks on it."[11]

What is lacking are direct investigations both of performance in the role and of perceptions of the role-set by those who are being socialized, to determine how and in what way these attitudes (e.g., cynicism and humanitarianism) are manifested. Just how does the "cynical" medical student or nurse approach a patient? Does the jaundiced view of the world, which cynicism implies, affect the motivation to perform, the perception of patients, or one's interest and concern?

In this study we are able to deal only with the student nurse's perception, not with her actual nursing role performance. What we did was to place that perception in particular interactional contexts which are relevant to role performance. Rather than obtaining measures on some general scale purporting to reveal the degree of cynicism, idealism or whatever, we chose to look at the students' responses to a relatively ambiguous stimulus—a photograph depicting a hospital scene—to which they would respond by writing an open-end free-response story. Thus the data we obtained represented the students' own perceptions of relevant situations, not responses to closed-end, pre-constructed questionnaires, or scales which embody assumptions of what constitutes humanitarianism or idealism. By analyzing these responses and determining content patterns, we

---

[11] Becker *et al., op. cit.,* pp. 420–421.

hoped to discover meaningful configurations that would enable us to say something about the manner in which the students' attitudes were expressed and how they changed. These changes could then be interpreted for their significance in relation to the concepts of idealism, realism, humanitarianism and cynicism. Our position was similar to that of Becker in that we did not view cynicism and idealism as general traits. We were looking at the expression of these and other attitudes in particular situational contexts as manifested by students who were involved in learning a new role. The expressions they manifested were relevant in terms of this role and not necessarily in terms of all their roles, that is to say, they may have shown idealism in one context at one time but not in another context at another time. Further, we wanted to interpret the meaning of these expressions and any changes in them from freshman to senior year. It is our position that "realism" or "realistic" attitudes may reflect the degree of the individual's socialization into the routine aspects of the role so that what was once novel and strange becomes commonplace and ordinary, i.e., part of the everyday rather than the unusual. In the course of learning a role, the individual learns how to normalize events and make them understandable. This is not to say that the normalization produces a desirable or even accurate interpretation of what is occurring. What it means is that to be able to grasp the meaning of events, the individual must fit them into a perspective that "makes sense" to him. Once having done so, he can then know what to do about them.

In the course of socialization, one learns how to do this easily and quickly, so that events that formerly seemed complicated, mysterious and incomprehensible become simplified, clarified and understandable. The expression and description of their simplicity can then seem to be callous, stereotyped, cynical, hard or any number of things. Alternatively, one who is able to perform such transformations can also be said to be "one who knows the situation," grasps it in its complexity and reduces it to those features most salient to the performance of the role.

In this analysis, therefore, we were searching for an interpretation of the changes which occurred as freshmen became seniors and of the differences between freshmen and seniors that were, on the one hand, consistent with notions of realism and humanitarianism, but which also embodied the situational relevance of the expression of an attitude. The context of situational relevance was taken to include not only the particular stimulus question or scene that the respondent reacted to but also who the respondent was, what she was becoming, and how that self was involved in the interpretation she made.

The Role Projective Test (RPT) developed by Albert Wessen consists of a set of ten photographs (slides) depicting a student nurse in a number of typical hospital situations. The photographs were taken in a hospital but actors rather than real patients or nurses were posed. They show the nurses on the ward in interaction with patients, a visiting physician, intern, visitor and other nurses.*

We used six of the ten slides in our study. They were projected on a screen for four minutes each to groups of student nurses. Instructions were given for each nurse to write a brief (10–12 lines) story about each picture as she saw it, giving not only a description of what was taking place, but also including some indication of the events that led up to the situation and the probable outcome of the situation depicted. The use of imagination in writing these stories was stressed.

The use of projective techniques by sociologists and anthropologists for purposes other than the study of individual personalities is still consistent with the general definition of projection, namely, ". . . a normal process whereby the individual's inner states or qualities influence his perception and interpretation of the outer world."[12] Projective tests which are designed to determine how various role performers perceive different roles are likely to present more structured stimuli, ask for a more limited range of responses, and be more specific and limited in their application than the traditional psychological projective tests devised for clinical purposes.[13]

---

* The visitor slide was omitted from the analysis because the content of stories was so distinctive that grouping was not possible. Since there was only one slide involving this situation interpretations based on it would be less reliable. The slides depicting interaction with other nurses were not included in the analysis reported here.

[12] Lindzey, G., *Projective Techniques and Cross-Cultural Research,* Appleton-Century-Crofts, New York, 1961, p. 31.

[13] For examples of this kind of use of projective tests, see: Reissman, L. and Rohrer, J. H., *Change and Dilemma in the Nursing Profession,* G. P. Putnam, New York, 1957; Abdellah, F. G., Methods of Identifying Covert Aspect of Nursing Problems, *Nursing Research,* 6, 1957, pp. 4–23; Copeland, M. *et al.,* A Projective Technique for Investi-

They are most helpful when freedom and spontaneity of expression are desired, particularly in exploratory stages of research when the variety of attitudes and perceptions possessed by subjects is not known, when direct questions are likely to produce descriptions of personal attitudes and feelings, and when a set of limited alternatives or specific questions would prevent one from learning how subjects interpret, perceive and organize events portrayed in a situation.[14] It would be more difficult and perhaps more threatening for the subject to be asked, "How would you behave in the following situation?" than to be asked for a free response to the same situation portrayed in a photograph. Subjects find it easier to express themselves if they are not speaking explicitly about their own feelings and attitudes.

Seventy-six freshman nursing students, class of 1965, at the General Hospital School of Nursing took the Role Projective Test (RPT) in January, 1963. They had entered in September, 1962, and had been exposed to approximately 11 weeks of clinical experience in the hospital. The senior group consisted of 29 senior students of the class of 1963 who took the RPT in August, 1963, and the entire remaining group (49) from the class of 1965 who took the RPT for the second time in June, 1965, just prior to graduation.

The major dimensions that were developed and used to analyze the stories developed out of a reading of the stories. The following features were mentioned in most of the stories: who initiated the interaction; the roles attributed to persons shown in the slide; the reasons for occurrence of the interaction; the specific type of interaction which occurred; emotional expressions attributed to others and the reasons for these; statements which indicated model, appropriate, correct or ideal behaviors, thoughts, or feelings for nurses and which were attributed to the student nurse (or expressed in the third person) by the respondent; statements which indicated inappropriate, inadequate, or incorrect behaviors, thoughts, or feelings for nurses and which were attributed to the student nurse

gating How Nurses Feel about the Use of Authority, *Nursing Research, 4,* 1955, pp. 79–86; Sayles, L. R., Field Use of Projective Methods, *Sociology and Social Research, 38,* 1954, pp. 168–173; and Goldschmidt, W. and Edgerton, R. B., A Picture Study of Values, *American Anthropologist, 63,* 1961, pp. 26–47.

14 Selltiz, C. et al., *Research Methods in Social Relations,* Holt and Co., New York, 1959, pp. 285–287.

(or expressed in the third person) by the respondent; and, finally, the outcome of the interaction.

Each of the six slides was examined separately and the story, or protocol, was taken as the unit of analysis. A response that could be classified as falling on one dimension was tabulated only once under one of the sub-categories of that dimension, i.e., multiple coding was not done.*

Some of the dimensions and their sub-categories were cross-tabulated in order to determine thematic patterns in the stories.

Because of the exploratory nature of the analysis, we did not deem it desirable to separate the two senior groups in order to develop a set of categories with the cross-sectional samples that could then be checked or tested for stability with the longitudinal group comparisons. By increasing the number of observations for the senior group we hoped to discover patterns or trends that might otherwise be obscured. Ideally, two independent samples of freshmen and seniors would be taken, the first to be used in the development of the categories and the second in the testing of hypotheses concerning freshmen-senior differences.

In the analysis, the cross-sectional freshman-senior comparisons and the longitudinal comparisons were tabulated and examined separately. If the observed differences between the cross-sectional and longitudinal comparisons were not consistent, i.e., in the same direction, or if no difference greater than 10% between the freshmen and

---

* For example, assume that one dimension had five sub-categories. A protocol would be scored for only one of these sub-categories even though other sub-categories also appeared in the story. The decisions as to which of the categories to score was made in terms of the following criteria: 1) If one of the sub-categories was, in the judgment of the scorer, the predominant theme or focus of the story it would be scored. 2) If no single sub-category could be judged as a major theme or focus of the story then the first-mentioned category would be scored. For some dimensions, problems such as these did not occur because the sub-categories were mutually exclusive. For example, for the dimension "who initiated the interaction," four sub-categories were used: 1) the student; 2) the other person in the slide; 3) someone not shown in the slide; and 4) no mention of who initiated the interaction, or unable to determine. The sub-categories are described in the analysis when differences between the groups exist. Otherwise only a listing of the sub-categories is given.

the seniors occurred, then no further treatment of the data was made. If both comparisons were in the same direction and differences greater than 10% were found, then the protocols from both senior classes were added together (i.e., a total of 78). In the analysis we focused primarily on the differences between the freshmen and seniors, not on the similarities.

When the same subjects were included in a longitudinal comparison using a test re-test design, there was a built-in correlation between the responses of freshmen and seniors since the same individuals' responses are being compared. This operates against the hypothesis that different patterns will be found for freshmen as opposed to seniors. Inclusion of the cross-sectional groups provided a firmer basis for assessing differences between freshmen and seniors though change in the same individuals could be assessed only in the longitudinal design. When both longitudinal and cross-sectional comparisons were in the same direction, we concluded that there was a consistent pattern for the two classes in the same school.

The stories which are quoted here appear exactly as the respondent wrote them, i.e., grammar, spelling and punctuation were not corrected. We chose to do this rather than undertake to edit the stories, and by editing, introduce distortion. Stories were identified by the class of the respondent and her code number.

We classified the stimulus photographs according to the category of the role portrayed by the other person (as validated by the student's perception) ; e.g., if the other person in the photograph was intended to be an intern but the student saw him as an orderly, then this response was removed from those classified under the heading of "seen as intern." Although the slide was called the "intern slide," responses which did not conform to this perception were excluded. For the presentation of the results of the analysis, the slides were grouped in terms of the roles portrayed by the actors. Slides depicting male medical personnel (doctors, interns or residents) are considered together. (The numbers of the slides refer to the order in which they were presented to the respondents) .

STUDENT NURSE AND PATIENT

Two slides depicting a student nurse interacting with a patient were shown (slides 1 and 9). Two additional slides, 6 and 7, although not specifically showing a patient, could be included under this heading because stories constructed by respondents frequently made reference to patients. They are described separately, however.

In response to slide 9, freshmen tended to write stories which mentioned both positive and negative emotional characteristics of the patient, e.g., the patient was lonely, worried, afraid, angry, demanding, crabby, cooperative, grateful, happy. As the following examples from these stories indicate, such emotional responses were found for a variety of reasons.

> This man has been in bed for three weeks and is tired and bored with it all . . . (freshman) .

> . . . She leaves with him happy . . . She then goes to the nurse's station and records her patient's condition in the nurse's notes. It would probably be something like: "Seems to be fairly comfortable and is in good spirits" (freshman) .

More freshmen than seniors saw the student nurse as responding to these emotions and feelings of the patient in a manner indicative of concern and with an effort to give emotional support (25% freshmen vs. 15% seniors) . The descriptions of the freshmen tended to have an idealistic quality in that the nurse was seen as effective in responding to the emotional needs of the patient which means that she not only knew what to do but she did it and achieved, as an outcome, the resolution of the patient's problem.

> The patient had been quite a problem for the staff. No one was able to cope with him. He threw bed pans, pillows & anything else he could get his hands on. The student dreaded to even go in his room, but since she had been assigned to him that day it was necessary for her to do so. After being with him that morning she became aware that he needed help & she began to look into his background. She found that his wife was very domineering & that the man was quite mousy & home & in his business. Knowing this she set up a plan to help him during his stay, she gave him the emotional care he needed & he welcomed her visits and care (freshman) .

The seniors more frequently saw the situation as one involving simple technical or physical problems such as providing a glass of water for the patient; the nurse would be able to meet these easily and thus the patient was not seen as a complicated, emotionally

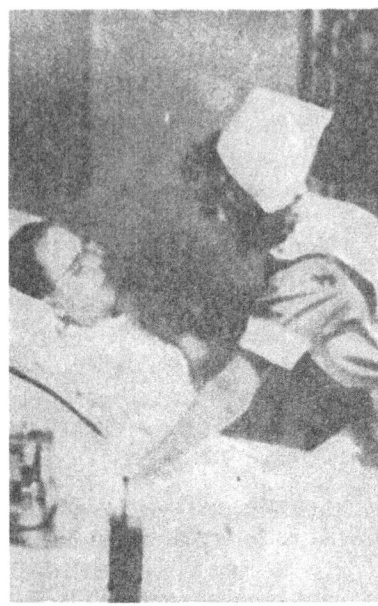

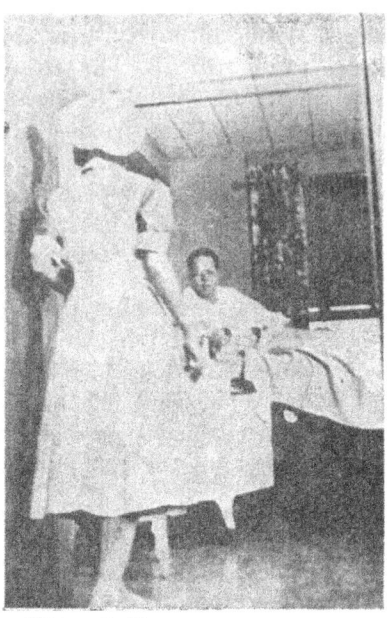

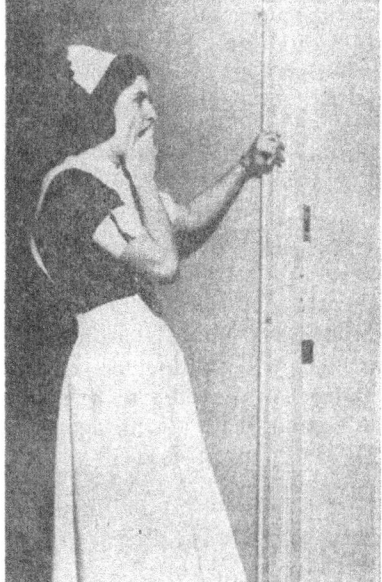

Upper Left

Slide 1. Student nurse is bending over patient who is reclining in hospital bed. She is holding a glass of liquid so that he can drink.

Upper Right
Slide 9. Student nurse is entering the door to patient's room. Patient is raised up in bed. He is holding the call buzzer in his right hand and is leaning and looking toward the door.

Left
Slide 6. Student nurse is standing in open doorway. Her hand is raised to her mouth, giving her an expression of shock, surprise, fear or amazement.

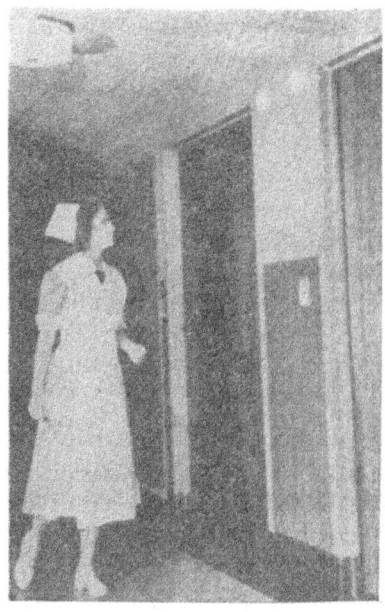

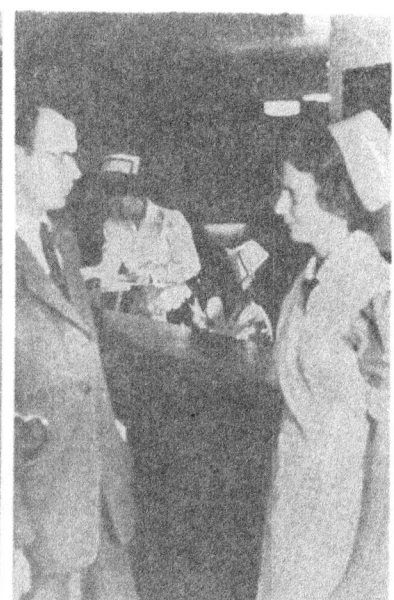

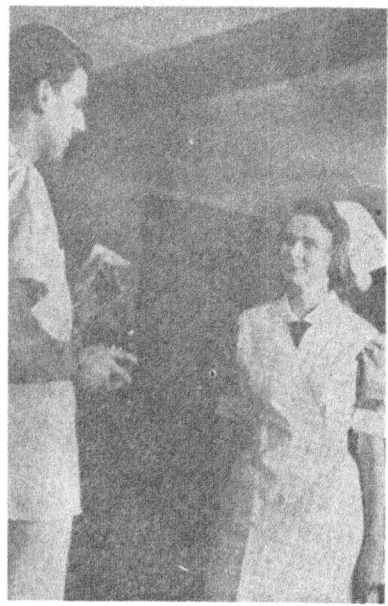

Upper Left
Slide 7. Student nurse is standing or walking in hospital corridor. She is looking up at what appears to be a call light on the wall between two doors.

Upper Right
Slide 3. Student nurse and doctor (in street clothes) are standing in front of the nurses' station. Two nurses are in the background.

Right
Slide 5. Student nurse stands in front of the nurses' station with her back to it. She is looking into the eyes of an intern who is standing in front of her holding a bottle half filled with some liquid.

reacting individual. For slide 9, this pattern was observed for 22% of the freshman stories and for 32% of the seniors'. For example:

> The patient called and the nurse went in to see what he wanted. He only wanted his bedpan emptied (senior).

Furthermore, the seniors more frequently than the freshmen described the situation in slide 1* in the simplest of technical terms. That is, proportionally more senior than freshman stories approximated a mere description of what was occurring in the picture, i.e., a nurse giving a patient a glass of water. Any "medical" implication to this activity merely involved offering medication with the glass of water or using the water in a minor therapeutic way, e.g., to quiet a cough or quench a thirst (30% freshmen; 46% seniors). For example:

> The nurse has properly prepared and poured a medication for this patient and is offering some water to wash it down. The effect of the medication on his condition will in time help better his condition (senior).

It seems then, that seniors have a greater tendency than freshmen to view the situation pictured in slide 1 as one in which a simple procedure is being carried out in a routine way or, alternatively, to present stories which are much more stimulus-specific with less imaginative elaboration.

If we were to interpret the different patterns and tendencies as reflections of changes occurring in the student over time, we would describe these changes as shifting from the freshman's description of the student nurse as a "model" student engaged in "appropriate," "correct," "Florence Nightingale-ish" behavior, thoughts or feelings, and who idealistically felt that situations ultimately end for the best, to the senior's description of the student nurse as one who was negligent or inadequate in her patient care, who engaged in unprofessional conduct, thoughts, or feelings, and who was negative or pessimistic in picturing the outcome of situations.

One indicator of this shift seemed to be revealed in the attitudes,

---

* This slide showed few differences between freshmen and seniors primarily because most descriptions referred to the event occurring in the slide. Therefore, slide 9 is the source of most of the data and discussion.

feelings and specific traits attributed to the student nurse. In response to slide 9, the freshmen were more likely than the seniors to describe the student as a "model" nurse using terms which, to them, connoted a "good" nurse—kind, tactful, understanding, sympathetic, efficient, pleasant (26% freshmen; 6% seniors).

In particular, the freshmen were more likely than the seniors to describe the student nurse as exhibiting this "model" behavior when confronted with a difficult patient who was demanding, crabby, irritable, angry, bored, lonely, disobeying orders, etc. (40% freshmen; 13% seniors). Occasionally this would involve an adaptation of what may be termed a "professional attitude," i.e., the inclinations of the nurse would be to avoid the patient or show irritation toward the difficult patient but, realizing that she is a nurse with certain professional duties and obligations, she would suppress her normal tendency and fulfill her professional responsibilities. This professional attitude was expressed somewhat more frequently by freshmen than seniors (16% freshmen; 5% seniors). For example:

> This patient had just turned on the call light at the nurses' station and this student nurse has come to answer it. The man is a chronic complainer and now he complains that he wants some fresh water. The nurse is disgusted with him, although she doesn't show it, because she just gave him fresh water 30 minutes ago. However, she cheerfully gets him what he wants (freshman).

Finally, in the construction of outcomes to the story, freshmen were found to be more "idealistic" than seniors who more frequently presented a "negative" outcome. In the responses to slide 9, this idealism was revealed in the tendency for a greater proportion of freshmen to construct outcomes which extol the accomplishments of the student nurse as adequately and successfully giving care to her patients (35% freshmen; 10% seniors). Furthermore, the freshmen more often portrayed the student nurse as being successful in adequately coping with the difficult patient (47% freshmen; 16% seniors). The freshmen were not only more idealistic in believing that situations in general turn out favorably, but their faith in the student nurse's ability was strong enough to lead them to believe that she could cope with even the very difficult patients. For example:

"Nurse! What has been keeping you? My breakfast tray is late. I need the bedpan, and I want to see my doctor." The patient is very demanding but the student remains calm and composed. She explains why the tray is late as she gives him the bedpan. Then she tells him the procedure he will follow, what to expect, when the doctor will see him, etc. She suspects that this patient is afraid, so she is tactful & kind to him. Gradually his gruff manner softens & he agrees to cooperate with her" (freshman).

Additional support for the interpretation that freshmen are more idealistic than seniors was found in the outcomes described. The freshmen were more likely than the seniors to state that as an outcome the "patient would (or did) recover" (slide 1: 22% freshmen; 7% seniors). The seniors, on the other hand, more frequently constructed an outcome with negative overtones in response to slide 9 (4% freshmen; 15% seniors). In the senior stories the student nurse was portrayed either as being unsuccessful in coping with emotional or physical needs of the patient or as being engaged in unprofessional conduct, thoughts, or feelings with regard to the patient. For example:

The man in the picture just had a relapse accompanied by much pain. The nurse is administering a drug to relieve him. He will recover fully from the medication given (freshman).

The patient is quite upset and combative. When the student starts to enter the room to help him with his bath, the pt. orders her out of the room and almost jumps out of bed. The student tries to reason with the patient unsuccessfully . . . (senior).

In summary, analysis of slides depicting nurse-patient interaction revealed two major differences between freshmen and senior student nurses in their care of and attitude toward patients and patient care. First of all, the freshmen tended to view the student nurse as being more "patient-centered" in her care of patients than did the seniors; the seniors tended to portray the student nurse as being more "technique centered" in her care of patients. The seniors' responses indicated that they would tend to give more perfunctory care to patients who have become "disease entities" rather than "whole" people with distinct personalities and that they would devote less energy than would freshmen toward viewing each patient as an individual whose needs must be met in a creative and distinctive fashion.

The second major difference was that freshmen were more idealistic than the seniors in their portrayal of the student nurse as a "model" student and in their construction of outcomes.

STUDENT NURSE ALONE

Slides 6 and 7 are similar in that both portray the student nurse by herself. The scene in slide 6 is not necessarily defined as a hospital setting, since only an open door is observed; whereas slide 7, in which a call light above the door is shown, is almost invariably seen as a hospital corridor.

These slides present relatively unstructured stimuli, thereby evoking freer use of imagination in the construction of stories. Nevertheless, two broad categories emerged in our analyses of students responses' to the situations depicted. One of these categories was directly related to the factor of experience as a nursing student while the other category was related to the theme of an idealistic portrayal of the student nurse.

Several separate findings reflected the inexperience of freshmen in nursing situations as compared to seniors. One fairly explicit indication of this was that, in their responses to slide 7, freshmen respondents more frequently described the student as someone who was "new" to a certain nursing situation or as someone who was doing something "for the first time" than did the seniors (37% freshmen; 10% seniors).

Another obvious indication of the relative inexperience of the freshmen as compared to the seniors was that freshmen, in response to slide 6, were more likely to portray the student as "calling for help" when faced with a situation which she thinks she cannot handle alone (26% freshmen; 13% seniors).

One of the nurses has sent the student to a room to pick up some equipment needed elsewhere.

Upon arriving at the room, the patient sees an immediate post-op patient sitting up in bed, having awakened and becoming frightened. She immediately calls for help . . . (freshman).

Another indicator of the relative inexperience of the freshmen was revealed in the description of reasons why the student nurse is standing in the hall in slide 7. Of those respondents who portrayed the student as going to see a patient, a larger percentage of freshmen than seniors depicted the student as "checking the patient's name and room number on the door" before entering to care for the patient (28% freshmen; 8% seniors), whereas a larger percentage of senior than freshman respondents depict the student as going to "answer a call light or call bell" without any mention of this checking routine (11% freshmen; 35% seniors). It was as if the freshmen, being new and unfamiliar with the hospital setting, were concerned with being properly oriented. This concern for orientation occurs whenever one enters a new situation, but it passes quickly and the factors in the environment are taken for granted by those who are familiar with the setting. Thus, the seniors, with greater experience, seldom made reference to a checking procedure.

The freshmen were more likely than the seniors to portray the student as reacting emotionally to the situation at the open door (72% freshmen; 49% seniors). Because many of these situations were also described by seniors but without any emotional response, the implication is that seniors treated these incidents in a more "matter-of-fact" way and no longer reacted emotionally.

Table 1 presents a tabulation of the students' descriptions of the situation shown in slide 6 and the frequency with which an emotional response by the student nurse depicted was described for each situation. Seniors were consistently lower in the frequency with

Table 1. Number and Percentage of Stories Attributing Emotional Reaction to Student Nurse by Topic of Story and Respondent's Year in School (Slide 6)

	Freshmen					Seniors				
	Emotional Reaction				Total,	Emotional Reaction				Total,
	Present		Absent			Present		Absent		
Topic of Story	N	%	N	%	N	N	%	N	%	N
Patient disobeyed doctor's orders	9	60.0	6	40.0	15	4	36.4	7	63.6	11
Patient fell out of bed or other mishap	6	75.0	2	25.0	8	4	40.0	6	60.0	10
Patient death or suicide (actual or threatened)	9	90.0	1	10.0	10	9	69.3	4	30.7	13
S.N made clinical error	4	100.0	–	–	4	2	50.0	2	50.0	4
Other situation	27	69.2	12	30.8	39	19	47.5	21	52.5	40
Total	55	72.4	21	27.6	76	38	48.7	40	51.3	78

which they described an emotional reaction by the student nurse, either positive or negative.

Excerpts from stories describing some of these situations follow:

Situation Involves a Patient Who Has Died

This nurse's patient has just died as she was going in to check on him. This is the first such case for this young nurse and she doesn't know what to do or where to turn. She seems to be quite taken in and frightened by it . . . (freshman).

The call light went on and the nurse ran to the room. Upon reaching the room, the nurse found the patient half in the bed and partially on the floor. She saw much blood in the bed and on the patient. It was then determined that the patient had begun hemorrhaging and tried to get out of bed for help but had fallen and expired before he could get help (senior).

Situation Involves a Patient Who Has Fallen Out of Bed or Been Involved in Other Mishaps

The nurse in this picture has been asked to come to a patient's room. The picture shows her standing shocked at the door—she is shocked because the patient on complete bedrest is lying sprawled on the floor . . . (freshman).

A student nurse stops almost in the door way of a patient's room. As she looks inside she sees him fall on the floor. She immediately thinks of a possible injury & also the accident report that she will have to fill out (senior).

Situation Involves a Patient Who Is Disobeying Doctor's Orders

Apparently the nurse is returning to her pt. that she had just left a few minutes ago. It looks like she is horrified at what she sees. The pt. probably wasn't supposed to be out of bed and has gotten out of bed and doing something he isn't supposed to be doing . . . (freshman).

Nursing student is taking care of a patient on complete bedrest who has a cardiac problem. As she enters room she finds him climbing over side rails. She quickly puts him back to bed, restrains him, reports incident & takes vital signs (senior).

In addition it should be noted that the freshmen were more likely than seniors to depict the student as experiencing negative emotional reaction in response to slide 6 (34% freshmen; 22% seniors). These negative emotions included such feelings as fear, nervousness, worry, unhappiness, horror, embarrassment and guilt. In contrast to other negative emotions, such as dislike or hatred of certain aspects of nursing, which directly indicate a certain degree of dissatisfaction with the profession and which probably increase with experience, these negative feelings do not necessarily connote dissatisfaction, but they seem to have an inverse relationship to the factor of experience as a nursing student.

Similarly, in response to slide 7, the freshmen more frequently than seniors described the student as experiencing fear or confusion, or as being timid and unsure (39% freshmen; 19% seniors).

In response to slide 6, the freshmen were more likely than the seniors to exhibit one or more of the negative emotions cited above when confronted with the following situations: a patient who has died; a nude patient; or a patient who had fallen out of bed or has been involved in some other mishap while in the hospital.

Finally, slide 7 provided further support for the conclusion that inexperience is directly related to the negative emotions which are attributed to the student nurse. This inexperience need not be measured by the respondent's year in school. If, instead of using the length of time in the school as our criterion, we consider all those stories which referred to the student as a "freshman" or as "doing something for the first time," we would find that a higher percentage of the stories also attributed some negative emotion to the student nurse than did those which specifically indicated that she was more experienced (e.g., a senior) or which did not mention her amount of experience.

Another difference between freshmen and seniors was that a larger percentage of freshmen depicted the student as possessing the attributes of a "model," "dedicated" and "idealistic" nurse. In contrast, the seniors were more likely than the freshmen to portray the student nurse as more oriented to the "world outside of nursing" and as less "idealistic."

In response to slide 6, the freshmen more frequently wrote statements which could be categorized as expressions of "idealized nursing role behavior" (17% freshmen; 1% seniors). These statements seemed to indicate that the respondent was perhaps reiterating what she had been taught (i.e., how a "good" or "successful" nurse would or should behave in such and such a situation) ; or that she was portraying her own conception of "good" or "successful" nursing behavior. If the student was depicted as performing poorly in the present situation, but the respondent either wrote that the student would excel in the future or admonished the student for her "inappropriate" or "incorrect" behavior, then these stories were also included as an expression of "idealized nursing role behavior." In other words, the student was either portrayed as a "model" nurse in the present situation or there was an idealistic belief that she would become one. The following quotation will demonstrate more clearly the specific nature of these statements:

> The nurse walks up to a door of a room & looks in before entering. She sees a sight that startles & shocks her. She stops & gasps. Undoubtedly she will recover hurriedly and enter the room. If the situation needs correcting she will do so in a calm, correct, formal & polite manner . . . (freshman) .

The seniors, on the other hand, were more likely than the freshmen to construct stories in response to slide 6 which specifically dealt with the non-nursing situation of heterosexual relationships (1% freshmen; 18% seniors) .

> Student goes in to assist doctor & another student for a procedure. They didn't know she was coming. He was kissing the other student. Result girl at the door was surprised & upset. She likes him too (senior) .

The results of our analysis of personality need scores, based on the Edwards Personal Preference Schedule administered to the same freshmen and seniors in the longitudinal study (see Chapter 5) , showed that the heterosexuality need increases significantly and to an extent greater than in non-nursing age-control groups. The stories seniors constructed were consistent with this pattern of growing interest in heterosexual activities.

The freshmen were more likely than the seniors to construct what was categorized as a "positive" outcome in response to slides 6 and 7, whereas the seniors were more likely than the freshmen to construct what was categorized as a "negative" outcome.

Positive outcomes included such statements as: "the patient recovers"; "the student will do a good job"; "the student gains confidence in her own ability"; "the student will learn how to handle the situation in the future"; "fortunately no harm developed from the student's error"; "the student enjoys her work and is in good spirits." In other words, positive outcomes were manifestations of an optimistic orientation which expressed the belief that situations turn out for the best in the end.

Negative outcomes included such statements as: "the patient dies"; "the student will not give adequate or proper patient care"; "the student is unhappy'"; "the student nurse is angry at, or dislikes, the patient." In these stories, the closure was, therefore, either pessimistic in its orientation, was representative of an "unprofessional" attitude of the student, or it indicated that the student was not a successful or model nurse.

We can conclude that two distinct freshman-senior differences appeared in the analysis of the slides portraying the student nurse alone in an undefined nursing situation. One of these differences reflected the relative inexperience of freshmen. It can be taken for granted that freshmen are less experienced than seniors, but the manner in which amount of experience affects a student's thoughts, feelings and behavior is not necessarily known. Stories written in response to these slides seem to indicate that the inexperienced student will be frightened, upset, nervous, embarrassed, and unsure of herself in performing and experiencing what will eventually become normal nursing tasks and events. She will be more likely to call for supportive assistance when unable to handle situations. She will check and recheck herself even before doing the simplest of tasks. These reactions, in all probability, are not only typical of the freshman student nurse but of novices in other fields as well.

Closely related to the factor of experience are other patterns. A novice may be typified as being highly motivated to do her best and as having aspirations of eventually becoming an outstanding worker. She is also inclined to have an optimistic orientation about life in general. Both patterns are found for freshmen more frequently than for seniors.

DOCTORS AND INTERNS

Slide 3 shows a physician, identified clearly by a stethoscope, and a student nurse standing in front of the nurse's station; this slide will be referred to as the "doctor slide." Slide 5 pictures a student nurse and a young man, dressed in a white hospital shirt and white trousers, standing in front of the nurse's station. The young man's age appears to range from twenty-five to thirty years. The combination of his age and dress result in an ambiguous definition of his exact position on the hospital staff. He was usually described by our subjects as an intern and for this reason the slide will be called the "intern slide." Occasionally, he was seen as a medical student, technician or orderly.

One basic distinction that can be made in how the relationship between the student nurse and the physician or intern is depicted is in terms of an instrumental or social-emotional focus. Instrumental relationships are those describing task and work and behavior relevant to the work aspects of the roles depicted. A social-emotional focus, on the other hand, refers to behavior oriented to expressing needs, emotions, and feelings whether overtly or in fantasy. Responses to persons depicted are not primarily oriented to their work roles though social-emotional expression can be seen as developing out of the instrumental aspects of task performance. The terms we have chosen to characterize these relationships are "professional" and "social."

The doctor slide was most frequently described as one in which relationships are strictly professional. For example:

This nursing student has just been on TPC (total patient care). The Dr. has just arrived & is asking about the pt. Perhaps something has just happened to the pt. or an unusual observance has been made. The nurse will report to the Dr. anything she feels he should know & they will proceed to the pt's room for examination & further observation (freshman).

For the intern slide, the interaction was seen as including a social relationship in addition to (or in place of) the professional relationship. For example:

The student heard that an intern she was dating would be working on her division. He comes up there needs help with a procedure and asks her to help. She must act & look professional even though she feels extremely awkward. They both act professional while the nurse assists the intern and later discuss it on their date that evening (senior).

A comparison of the stories of freshmen and seniors showed

that a smaller proportion of seniors than freshmen described the relationship depicted in the doctor slide as strictly professional, but that there was little difference between their responses to the intern slide. The perception of the interaction depicted in the intern slide as involving only a professional relationship is considerably lower than for the doctor slide. Again, seniors were somewhat more likely to see only social relationships occurring, whereas freshmen, if they did describe these as present, also saw professional relationships simultaneously. (*See* Table 2). Therefore, it appears that both the male's age and his status in the hospital hierarchy affected the type of relationship the student nurse saw. The closer he was in age and status to the student nurse, the more likely she was to perceive the possibility of social relationships in their interaction.

Turning to the specific characteristics of the student nurses' descriptions of the professional relationship with physicians and with interns, it was found that this professional relationship varied, depending on the male's position in the hospital hierarchy, and that there was a further difference which seemed related to the student's year in nursing school. The freshmen were more likely than the seniors to view their professional contact with physicians as placing the student in the role of an "information-giver." In most instances, they indicated that it would be the physician, knowing

Table 2. Number and Percentage of Stories for Professional and Social Relationships Described by Respondent's Year in School for Slides 3 and 5

	Doctor Slide (3)				Intern Slide (5)			
	Freshmen		Seniors		Freshmen		Seniors	
Type of Relationship	N	%	N	%	N	%	N	%
Professional	75	98.7	67	87.0	24	32.9	20	27.0
Social	–	–	9	11.7	17	23.3	25	33.8
Professional and social	1	1.3	1	1.3	32	43.8	29	39.2
Total	76	100.0	77[a]	100.0	73[a]	100.0	74[a]	100.0

[a]Although there were 76 freshman and 78 senior stories, in some the man's position on the hospital staff was left unstated or, as happened in one senior's story, the physician was seen as "a visitor."

that nurses and even student nurses have frequent contact with his patients, who would approach her seeking information about his patient's condition:

> This student's patient is also the doctor's patient. He is getting ready to go see his patient. He wants to know how his patient is getting along. When he asked the head nurse she referred him to the student who is taking care of the patient. The student is telling him that his patient feels much better this a.m. . . . (freshman) .

Seniors, on the other hand, were somewhat more likely than freshmen to view the physician as teaching the student about his patient's condition, or about some aspect of patient care, or discussing other medically related matters. In most of these teaching situations the student, being curious or concerned about her patient or some aspect of his care, would initiate the interaction by directly approaching the physician:

> This student is quite concerned about her patient's prognosis—she has a chance to find out for she has spotted his doctor. She is asking about her patient . . . (senior) .

Although one would suspect that freshmen might have been more apt to view the physician as a teacher, it may be that freshmen considered the physician too busy to take time out to instruct a student nurse. In other words, the freshmen seemed to view their role vis-a-vis the physician as being of service to him as an information-giver rather than as his being of service to them as a teacher.

The freshmen were more likely than the seniors to point out the importance of the role of the nurse in the patient-nurse-physician relationship (30% freshmen; 5% seniors) . The function of a nurse as an information-giver was seen as "essential" or "important" because of the resultant increase in the physician's knowledge of his patient's condition which "enables him to give better care to his patient." A few freshmen also saw the role of student nurse as essential or important because she may serve as a "check" on the physician by "catching his mistakes," or because "he will work better with the nurse at his side." It was as if the freshmen possessed an elaborate idealistic notion about the nursing profession which would almost disappear by their senior year.

Freshmen also tended to perceive the results of professional contact with physicians in more idealistic terms than did seniors. For the freshmen, this type of interaction situation would end with some type of improvement in the medical or nursing staff and with ultimate improvement in patient care (59% freshmen; 32% seniors). Primarily, this improvement was made possible by the student's functioning as an information-giver, thereby enhancing the physician's knowledge of his patient's condition.

The professional relationship which students have with interns* (or residents or medical students) was seen as different from their professional relationships with physicians.† Very few freshmen or senior nursing students portrayed the intern as a teacher, and only a few freshmen portrayed the student as an information-giver. Freshmen primarily viewed the intern as someone who asked the nurse to perform some simple technical activity for him—most frequently this would consist of taking a specimen to the laboratory. Seniors most frequently viewed the intern as also asking the student to assist him but usually in a more complicated nursing procedure. Finally, some seniors and some freshmen portrayed the intern as having less experience in the particular hospital setting (i.e., the intern was new on the ward) than the student and as asking for her guidance.

In contrast, data from the doctor slide indicated that physicians were never portrayed as asking for guidance from the students.

He is a new intern and is asking the student where the equipment can be found. He has been asking questions all morning. She will go and show him where everything is and then go with him & help him c the procedure (senior).

---

* For purposes of this analysis, all respondents who identified the young man as an orderly or technician were not included, since their position in the hospital status hierarchy was so much lower than interns, residents and medical students.

† The differences between the professional relationship students have with physicians, on the one hand, and with interns (or residents or medical students) on the other hand, must be interpreted with caution due to the nature of the two slides. The fact that the intern had a bottle in his hands, while the physician had a stethoscope in his pocket but was holding nothing in his hands may have influenced the content of their "professional" interaction.

Such stories reflect the realities of hospital life. Interns come and go and, when new on the ward, they need to find out where things are and what the routine is. The staff physician, on the other hand, has generally been there longer than the student nurse.

With regard to the outcome of the interaction, freshmen and seniors both tended to view the outcome of their professional contacts as resulting in an ultimate improvement in the ability of physicians and nurses to administer care to their patients.

With regard to social relationships, three major categories appeared. One was the description of a platonic relationship such as would exist between friends of the opposite sex. In other words, there would be no implication that the two people had a romantic interest in each other or a dating relationship. For example:

This is apparently a picture of an intern and a student nurse. The doctor is nice and kids around with the student nurse. The student seems to like the doctor and she thinks what he said was pretty funny. He told her he has a fly trapped in this bottle (freshman).

A second type of social interaction was seen in descriptions of the student as having a "crush" on the physician or intern which was not being reciprocated (or was not mentioned as being reciprocated). Occasionally, the explanation for his lack of reciprocation would be the discovery by the student that he was already married. In other stories, there would be no reciprocation, but the mere fact that he would say "Hello" or speak to her would be satisfying to the student. An example of such a non-reciprocal "crush" relationship is:

The young intern wants someone to clean his equipment up for him. The young S. N. seems to have a crush on the intern so she "dutifully" volunteers for the unwanted job. The Dr. is briefing her on exactly what he wants done & is being very explicit about it. The S. N. is supposedly paying close attention to him but instead her mind is wandering while she's thinking what a nice husband he'd make. The outcome will be that the S. N. will do the job, but afterwards she'll find out that the Dr. is already married & has two children (freshman).

The third type of social interaction described was the possibility or actual occurrence of a reciprocal romantic relationship, whereby either the student was dating or had an opportunity to date the intern or physician. Some implied that the romantic interest was (or would become) mutual.

This reciprocal relationship was normally restricted to an actual or eventual dating relationship. Only one senior in response to the doctor slide mentioned that the student and physician were married, and this was a secret marriage:*

> The nurse admired this doctor. They are secretly married but it is against the rules. This is an unexpected meeting in the halls. Both are trying to act very casual because the R.N.'s in the background might report them. They will talk briefly and then depart (senior).

A few seniors, however, explicitly or implicitly incorporated an element of promiscuity in their reciprocal relationship with the intern (8%) and with the physician (5%). This promiscuity consisted primarily of going out with the intern or physician even though he was married, or "having an affair" with him:

> The nurse has just told the M. D. about a dream she had of the 2 of them. He makes a proposition. She accepts (senior).

> The student and the intern are discussing what time she can sneak into his room tonight. They are both married (not to each other) so that makes it difficult. But the affair will crystalize (senior).

It was difficult to make meaningful comparisons between the kinds of social interactions described for the doctor slide and the intern slide since so few respondents saw the student nurses as being involved in social relationships with physicians.† However, one

---

* At the time this test was administered to this senior respondent, it was against the school regulations for nursing students to be married during the three year training period except during the last five months of their senior year.

† Since the male's status in the hospital setting would not normally be expected to affect the type of social relationship in the same way that a professional relationship would be affected, orderlies and technicians were grouped with interns, medical students and residents for this analysis.

noticeable difference was the absence of reference to any platonic relationship between the student nurse and the physician. Another difference was that when a social relationship was described for the doctor slide, it was more likely to be a reciprocal romantic or dating relationship. The following example is from slide 3 protocols:

> The doctor saw the student last night. He is asking if she got into the dorm all right so late at night. Student states two other students saw her. They will talk! (senior).

Since only one freshman described a social relationship with the physician, it was impossible to make any freshmen-senior comparisons other than to note that it was the seniors who were more likely to perceive this type of interaction between students and physicians.

There was no freshman-senior difference between the types of social relationships student nurses had with interns (or medical students, residents, technicians or orderlies in slide 5). However, when the distinction was made between those whose status in the hospital setting was higher than that of the student nurse (i.e., interns, residents and medical students) and those of equal or lower status than the student nurse (i.e., orderlies and technicians), a freshmen-senior difference emerged. Only the seniors saw the student as interacting socially with orderlies and technicians. Nine of the 57 senior respondents (16%) who described social relationships saw the young man as a technician or orderly. Of these nine, six (66%) viewed the relationship as a romantic rather than a platonic one. Perhaps this result may be interpreted as a more realistic approach on the part of seniors concerning the possibility for romantic relationships with men on the hospital staff. It has been hypothesized that the opportunity to have a social relationship with, and eventually to marry, a man in the medical profession is an expectation of many girls who enter nursing. Some from lower socioeconomic backgrounds may expect to be able to achieve upward social mobility by marrying physicians. The stories written by these nurses permit the inference that student nurses are oriented to the possibility of social dating relationships with men on the hospital staff and often see this as a very desirable and attractive possibility. However, it may be that by the time one becomes a senior, such relationships with orderlies and technicians, who are of lower or equal status, are more realistic expectations.

Further evidence of the seniors' tendency to view the romantic-social relationship in a more realistic, or what might also be termed a more mature fashion was revealed in the manner in which the student's interest in the young man was stated. Freshmen were more likely to depict the student as experiencing emotional feelings which resembled the typical high-school "crush." Not only did the freshmen more frequently indicate that the student had a "crush" on the young man (69% freshmen; 44% seniors), but they were also more likely to depict the student as experiencing satisfaction by merely being around or being noticed by him (39% freshmen; 8% seniors). Conversely, the seniors were more likely to depict a romantic or dating relationship as occurring (56% seniors; 31% freshmen). The implication would be that the seniors were more accustomed to the idea of having romantic or dating relationships with men on the hospital staff. This difference can best be demonstrated by the following examples from freshman and senior responses:

The student nurse assisted the intern with starting I.V. fluids. Now there in the corridor talking and he is thanking her for helping him. The patient will receive his fluids the nurse will be flying on a cloud being able to assist the most handsome intern and the intern will be busy about his other duties (freshman). (Non-reciprocated romantic crush; satisfaction from mere contact.)

This intern is conversing with the S. N. They are both working nights. They are planning a date for the next Saturday night, since they have that day off. They are going dining (cheaply) & either dancing or playing cards with a few other couples. They will both enjoy themselves (senior). (Reciprocal dating relationship; no strong evaluative or emotional terminology.)

The results of the analysis of responses for the doctor and intern slides (3 and 5 respectively) revealed that students viewed their relationships with physicians in a different manner than their relationships with interns (medical students, orderlies or technicians) and that these relationships changed as the student advanced in school. Most of the changes that occurred between freshman and senior year seemed to reflect the older age and increased experience of the seniors. In other words, as the student approached twenty-one (the average age of most senior nursing students in a diploma program) she was more likely to perceive herself as having social relationships with older physicians as well as with the younger interns, medical students, orderlies and technicians.

Her three years of education and experience enable the student to perform more complicated nursing procedures for physicians and interns. In addition, this experience enables her to see that a student's role vis-a-vis the physician does not place her almost exclusively in the position of being of service to the physician as an information-giver. Rather, the senior recognizes that the physician may also be relied on as a teacher, thereby indirectly being of service to the student.

With the increase in age and experience the student also comes to view these professional and social relationships, with their resultant consequences, more realistically. In the professional relationship with physicians she is less likely to possess idealistic conceptions about how essential her role is in the patient-nurse-physician relationship. Furthermore, she is less likely to possess a naive optimism that professional contact with physicians results in an ultimate improvement in the ability of physicians and nurses to administer care to their patients.

The same quality of optimism pervades the freshman's description of social relationships and romantic interests. In contrast, the seniors show what can again be characterized as realism. Descriptions of sexual interest and fulfillment are matter of fact—they simply occur and the parties involved are open-eyed, not starry-eyed. Mere co-presence is not sufficient to provide satisfaction for the senior and it is the seniors, older and more knowledgeable concerning life in the hospital, who assist interns, orient them and date them—even physicians are possible romantic targets who may reciprocate the interest shown. The romantic and social relationships described by freshmen are interesting in that they include descriptions of involvements with medical staff which persist through the senior year. The fact of their being eligible young girls with strong sexual interests is not a transitory phenomenon. In fact, those who remain into the senior year represent a group whose numbers have already been depleted by marriage. That sexual interests exist cannot be doubted. What is striking is the pervasiveness of this theme in the hospital setting.

Sexual behavior has not been systematically studied in occupational or job settings, but it is obvious that in some settings greater opportunities may be available, with high interest and receptiveness on the part of co-workers, due to the presence of large numbers of eligible young persons. The student nurse is not only in a setting in which young, desirable men may be found (nurses do sometimes marry doctors) but she is also in the more restrictive setting of the school of nursing. Thus, she often finds her every activity subject to scrutiny, and her outside social activities often being reported to her instructors and counselors. This setting is more restrictive than that of college, particularly the co-educational college, where dating is a major activity.[15] As a nurse in training, her attitudes, morals manners, mode of dress, speech, grooming and habits are all subject to inspection and sanction. The fantasies of romantic involvement can be interpreted as "escape," but the seniors' more realistic descriptions of meeting, dating and having affairs with doctors or interns and with technicians or orderlies represent both a response to the restrictive environment of the school and an orientation to the general age and sex roles in which they find themselves. In these stories, the greater frequency with which a non-professional or non-instrumental theme is described indicates greater diffuseness in attention to the situation depicted. The tasks being performed are less situationally specific and the possibility of non-work relevant behavior occurring under the cover of work is not doubted. Freshmen and seniors are both aware of these possibilities. In Chapter 7 figures are presented concerning the frequency with which these girls married doctors.

Being a nurse, then, includes the ability to integrate activities, such as those of sociability, with the performance of nursing tasks. In this area of activity, the seniors may not have any advantage over the freshmen since this type of overlapping of activities is

---

[15] Fox, D. J. and Diamond, L. K., *Satisfying and Stressful Situations in Basic Programs in Nursing Education,* Bureau of Publications, Teachers College, Columbia University, New York, 1964, report that incidents described by students indicated that the atmosphere of the school and the hospital was perceived as having a strong authoritarian component. Students wrote of being treated as adolescent girls by most school regulations, while at the same time, mature and responsible behavior was expected of them in the hospital. The most frequent complaints concerned the rigidity of residence regulations.

something that can be learned and practiced in other settings as well. That is, flirting, making dates, and engaging in double entendre conversation is rehearsed by females and males in this society through the high-school years and even before. Seniors are different from freshmen in the extent to which they conceive of the successful culmination of such activities or in the lowered (and in our view, more realistic) aspirations they have concerning whom they can date and marry. Physicians and interns are older, have more years of education and tend to be married. They are almost out of range, and when one is found to be unmarried, it is a pleasant surprise. What is realistic, then, if an affair of the heart is to be consummated, is to meet clandestinely and to set one's aspirations accordingly. The meaning of this kind of realistic orientation is similar to that already described. Our respondents were telling us what happens, what is possible and what the likely outcomes are. The persistence of stories describing romantic "crushes" differed in the extent to which seniors found these to be satisfying (fewer seniors than freshmen). Sex and romance continue to be important for seniors, but consummation, rather than satisfaction in fantasy, is sought.

DISCUSSION AND INTERPRETATION

In general, these results do show that in the variety of role relationships and situations depicted in the Role Projective Test, freshmen expressed a degree of idealism and optimism not found among seniors. Freshmen also showed greater concern with problems and difficulties of nursing practice, with relationships with patients and with problems faced in nursing school. However, their optimism pervaded such encounters and their stories depicted outcomes in which progress, satisfactory results and favorable outcomes occurred.

In relation to patients, seniors gave more technique-oriented than patient-centered care, viewed patients more as "disease entities" than "whole" people with distinct personalities, and devoted less energy toward meeting patient needs in a creative and distinctive fashion. The freshmen saw the student nurse as a "model" student and depicted favorable outcomes.

In situations that are relatively undefined, i.e., student nurse alone, the less experienced freshmen saw themselves as frightened, nervous, upset, embarrassed and unsure of themselves in performing and experiencing what eventually would become normal nursing tasks. Despite their insecurities, however, they not only aspired to succeed but described outcomes in which problems were resolved.

In relation to physicians and residents, some of the stories reflect the growth of interest in heterosexual activities on the part of seniors. Seniors are less likely to have "crushes" and more likely to have "affairs." The realities of the status differences between themselves and physicians and residents enter into the seniors' perceptions of social interaction with orderlies and technicians (the same persons who were previously seen as interns).

With increased experience in the hospital, the senior was less likely than the freshman to describe the student nurse as a valuable contributor to the physician in providing better patient care.

The patterns described in these results showed a striking consistency. Youthful idealism and optimism gave way to a realism based on experience, adaptation to the nursing role and to changed definitions of the situation.

Questions can be raised concerning the meaning of these changes. Is it possible that idealistic views represent perceptions of the role which outsiders, because they cannot know what it is to be in the role, bring with them? Experience in the role rather than didactic teaching about the role produces changed perceptions and, in a sense, a restructuring of the phenomenal world of the actor. The freshman or neophyte has only the definition of the role, as it is presented in didactic teaching or popular attitudes, to base her perception on; however, with experience, things are not the same as they were because the individual is no longer the same. She cannot perceive things in the same way because she has changed. She has come to know what it means to be an actual self, not merely an imagined self in the situation. Her first few performances have not yet enabled her to achieve the internal reorganization of perception and understanding of the world-as-it-is. Obviously, if only a few experiences were all that is needed to achieve this, the teaching of adequate role-performance and the reorganization of a self in relation to that role would be easily accomplished. But even longer term incumbents of a role do not all necessarily perceive the world (i.e., the particular role-set in question) in identical fashion.

Formal training and education do not in and of themselves operate to produce such changes. Our understanding of the reshaping of the individual—of the production of a new self—is not adequate yet to permit us to say *how* this is achieved. We know that for some students it never occurs, but for others it occurs to the extent that experts in the socialization of the neophyte may say "Now, there's a real ———" (substitute for the blank space the name of whatever role is being taught).

In short, we are proposing an alternative interpretation of the meaning of "idealistic" or "realistic" attitudes as they concern the role. Rather than assigning motivational significance to them, or regarding them as factors which affect performance, we can view them as indicators of the extent of socialization, i.e., the learning of the role. The learning we have in mind includes a cognitive orientation to the world of nursing which involves treating that world as it is, seeing in it what is, in fact, in it, and developing a perspective that is congruent with the perspectives of other relevant actors in the situation to the extent that all the actors can, in fact, successfully interact with one another.*

For example, the nurse who expects to find, on entering the patient's room, an emergency situation that she cannot cope with and which requires that she call for help, has a perspective that poses interactional dilemmas both for herself and others. The mere entry into a patient's room is normally a routine activity which contains perceivedly normal features.[16] By "normal" is meant those things which a socially competent actor can recognize, respond to, and deal with in a competent manner. There will be problems on occasion, but that which is defined as a problem is a "nursing problem" and therefore subject to a set of rules which normalize

---

* In some respects, this is consistent with the view of Becker *et al.,* who hold that the perspective of the actor must be viewed in the context in which it appears. It differs in emphasis in that expressions of realism or cynicism are seen as indicators of successful socialization and of the adoption of relevant perspectives rather than as situational adaptations. These perspectives *are* the subject's view, i.e., the real self, though that self may later change.

[16] For more complete discussions of the significance of the normalization of activity, discussions by Garfinkel and Schutz are relevant. The present discussion owes much to their work. Garfinkel, H., Studies in the Routine Grounds of Everyday Activities, *Social Problems, 11,* pp. 225–250, 1964; and Schutz, A., *The Collected Papers of Alfred Schutz, 1,* Martinus Nijhoff, The Hague, 1962.

it and make it manageable. For example, a nurse might enter a room and find a man, dressed in a patient's robe, painting the walls. If he is a patient, his painting activity can be normalized to mean that he is mentally disturbed and has to be treated as a psychiatric prob- lem; there are rules that prescribe how such a problem is to be handled. But suppose he is a painter who decided to put on patient's garb while painting the room. As a painter, his behavior, including his mode of dress, is not relevant to the nurse's performance of a nursing role vis-a-vis the other. He is not to be treated as a patient, but as a painter. Admittedly, he may be a strange painter, but his problematic behavior is not a nursing problem. One could declare, "Get that strange painter *out* of here"; whereas if he were a patient, one would be more likely to declare, "Let's put him *in* the psychi- atric ward." Nursing procedures would not prescribe how to deal with strange painters but they would prescribe how to deal with patients who act strangely.

Now the nurse who sees all kinds of possible unhandleable events occurring in patient rooms has not yet learned how to nor- malize the apparent problematic features of the scene. Freshmen, despite such unusual and trouble-filled descriptions, are neverthe- less socialized sufficiently to be able to say that the nurse *will* learn how to deal with these things in the future or that she will become a better nurse. What these remarks point to, it seems, is an aware- ness of the *existence* of knowledge and procedures concerning how to normalize events, though the student does not yet possess this knowledge herself. Not yet knowing what to do, she cannot confi- dently assert what to do. The expression of these "tales of fantasy" can also be interpreted to mean that the respondent is aware of her lack of relevant knowledge and skills. The sophisticated senior can ignore the occurrence of such events because they are no longer problematic. The problems she sees are not troubles in the sense of being situations for which prescribed rules may not yet be known or for which none exist. Instead, they are problems which involve performing according to standards within the limits of the role, e.g., how to perform all her duties within the time allotted, or how to remain kind and attentive despite her work load. Or, as many stories concerning interactions with patients show, there are no problems—activity is routine. To those of us who are outsiders, the merely routine attention to the patient and the lack of expressed concern for his emotional needs may appear to be a cynical ap- proach. For those in the role, the activity that is described may, in fact, be the one which is routinely performed and the approach the one which is most consistent with the performance of the other facets of the role. In short, it is routine daily activity. Stories that describe it are saying what is and, therefore, those who construct such stories are knowledgeable as to "the way things are." Whether it is a desirable state of affairs is another question. To learn how things are, we generally ask those who have been in the field for a long time. To determine how things *ought to be* is a matter on which neither neophytes nor old-timers are the final authority.

In contrast, idealism can be interpreted to mean that the neophyte is aware of her present limitations and can only express the hope and expectation that these will be overcome. Such stories may also serve a wish-fulfillment and anxiety-reduction function. But we prefer to interpret their significance for socialization as meaning that the emerging self is seen as competent rather than incompetent, that a belief exists that events can be normalized and that "what to do" will become known and routine although it may not be so at the moment.

This interpretation can be extended to the responses to the several slides used in our study. The realism, and what sometimes appears to be cynicism, concerning the nurse's tasks and duties and her interaction with patients, doctors and nurses, represents an awareness of events that can and do occur in the situations depicted. The senior responses show that situations that were formerly difficult and disturbing or were described as containing considerable diversity of activity, become routine, understandable and easily dealt with. Novelty has also worn off; the only area in which it seems to remain is that involving sexual activities. As the work situation becomes routine, it can also be expected to become less attractive to the practitioner. That this result could occur within three years and while the girl is still in school does not speak well for the development of an academic or professional interest or for an increased dedication to the role. The training program for nurses becomes, as Becker observed for medical school, something to "get through." Then an orientation to the world of work and to life-after-school begins to offer the new experience and novelty which was originally associated with entering school. The re-assertion of a new idealism, oriented toward the practice of nursing and the world of work and marriage, rather than school, can be expected, much as Becker found for the senior medical student.

Viewed in this way, a succession of new experiences, scheduled sequentially and step-wise so that successful achievement in one is a necessary prerequisite for entry into another, may be an effective way of maintaining the challenge held by new situations and the awareness of a need to develop skills to cope with them.* However, idealism, as expressed in optimism, hope and romanticized versions of what goes on in hospitals, is not to be interpreted as a motivational factor alone. Rather, such expressions can be assessed in terms of the extent to which they reflect the degree of learning of the role and the more realistic perception of life-as-it-is for those who perform the role as a routine daily activity.

It is our conclusion that the realistic perceptions of life-as-it-is which are held by these respondents and by other nursing and medical students who have been studied, is problematic for the professions only to the extent that the features of the world perceived by the student are judged to be undesirable. The student's perception cannot be localized as a phenomenon internal to the student and which is determined by individual characteristics. Such a judgment would lead to efforts to change the perceiving individual. Instead, the world-perceived may need to be re-structured so that the undesirable perceptions of it may also change. The dilemma with regard to strategies of change is that the individual's perceptions may harden into a set which affects subsequent perceptions of even changed situations. With specific reference to nurses, the early formation of perceptions and cognitive structurings of the world of nursing, in the fashion shown by third-year student nurses included in our study, makes subsequent re-socialization difficult. The implication is that the effective time for changing nurses is during the formal socialization period, i.e., while they are still in nursing school.

---

* I am grateful to Daniel V. Caputo for this suggestion.

Chapter 5

The Personality of the Student Nurse*

Results of several research projects show that entering nursing students are characterized by a distinctive set of personality needs; that several nursing student groups considered together show similar patterns for the years while in school; and that the effects of training show a consistent pattern of producing change in certain personality needs in directions opposite to or greater than those which would be expected from maturational effects. Further, training also operates to suppress changes in some personality needs and to enhance changes in others.

This chapter presents an analytic design and data relevant to understanding the relation between personality needs and the nursing role. Results of studies in which the Edwards Personal Preference Schedule, EPPS, was administered to nurses are collected and analyzed in order to determine what diploma school students are like.

In this chapter, we propose to set forth and apply, insofar as possible, an analytic design which can be used in studying the relation between personality and role. The design is intended to provide a broad framework to indicate how studies of personality, although done at different times and places, can be combined and compared.

---

* This chapter was written with the assistance of Jon Plapp.

Secondly, a number of studies already reported in the literature and new data from our own research are presented, within the framework of this design, to determine the degree of change and the time when, within the sequence of events leading from initial "choice" of an occupation to actual performance of the occupational role, distinctive personality characteristics exist or develop for nurses.

The problem of determining the relation between personality and occupational role has been the subject of much discussion by sociologists and psychologists. General discussions of the problem of determining the relationship between personality and social role or an occupational role as a type of social role are presented by Cohen, Merton, Parsons and Levinson.[1]

Sociologists, in general, have focused on such questions as the effect on the personality of employment in a particular type of institution or tenure in a professional role. Merton, Parsons and Levinson, as representatives of this orientation, tend to consider the problem when persons are beyond the training stage. Moreover, their discussions tend to be general and theoretical with little data presented which would show the manner in which the organization affects the individual personality. Studies of how individuals change over time, which are necessary to support these theories, are noticeably lacking. In general discussions, the assumption is often made that the characteristics shown by successful performers of an occupational role represent the combined effects of training, the institutional setting in which the role performer is found, and the demands of the role itself. Separating these various effects is recognized as an important task but nevertheless, little research has been undertaken in an effort to assess them.

Psychologists, on the other hand, have tended to study the dis-

[1] Cohen, Y., *Social Structure and Personality,* Holt, New York, Chapter 7, "Occupations and Professions," 1961, pp. 187–224; Merton, R. K., "Bureaucratic Structure and Personality" in *Personality in Nature, Society and Culture,* ed. by C. Kluckhohn, Knopf, New York, 1955, pp. 376–385; Parsons, T., "The Professions and Social Structure," in *Essays in Sociological Theory,* The Free Press, Glencoe, Illinois, 1949, pp. 34–99; and Levinson, D., Role, Personality and Social Structure in the Organizational Setting, *Journal of Abnormal and Social Psychology, 58,* 1959, pp. 170–180.

tinctive personality characteristics of successful occupational role performers.[2]

Super, in reviewing evidence from a variety of studies, concluded that:

> . . . personality traits seem to have no clear-cut and practical significant relationship to vocational preference, entry, success or satisfaction. . . . (but) if occupations are sufficiently narrowly and precisely defined, for example, in terms of functional specialties within an occupation, significant personality differences in occupational groups may be found. Perhaps some will be found which are so highly structured that only individuals with certain traits are successful or satisfied in them, whereas others will be found in which there is so little structure that individuals with greatly varying personality patterns can find satisfaction in them, each structuring the occupation in his own way. . . .

> In certain occupations, although not apparently in others, it is possible to construct a picture of the typical personality. (However) these personality sketches are not sufficiently clear cut to provide a scientific basis for occupational choice . . .[3]

Evidence for the existence of what might be called occupational personalities is found in the work of Roe who studied eminent men in various fields, e.g., biologists, psychologists, anthropologists and physical scientists.[4] Descriptions of the differences among the personalities of academic scientists are presented but it is not clear at what point in the development of the individual the distinctive elements in the personalities develop, or how training and/or subsequent performance in the role shape the personality.

Sociologists and anthropologists have assumed that a relation between personality and occupational role has been demonstrated. Within these theories, explicit recognition is given to the fact that

---

[2] The work of Roe, A., *The Psychology of Occupations,* New York, John Wiley & Sons, 1956; and Henry, W. E., The Business Executive: The Psychodynamics of a Social Role, *American Journal of Sociology, 54,* 1949, pp. 286–291, is relevant.

[3] Super, D., *The Psychology of Careers,* Harper, New York, 1957, p. 240.

[4] Roe, A., A Psychological Study of Eminent Psychologists and Anthropologists, and a Comparison with Biological and Physical Scientists, *Psychological Monographs, 67, 2,* 1953.

personality can change over time. It is not assumed that personality is determined at an early age and then "set" for life. It is possible that within the career stages found in occupations we would also find distinctive constellations of personality traits emerging and developing over time. Longitudinal studies would be extremely helpful in allowing us to assess the extent of change and pinpoint more precisely the points in time at which changes occur. With the selection of appropriate control groups, it would also be possible to determine to what extent changes are due to maturation, training and actual performance in the occupation.

The combination of sociological with psychological approaches blends into a distinctive social psychological orientation. We see the individual moving into a succession of roles each providing, to some extent, institutionalized definitions concerning behavioral expectations. As each stage is entered, some factors operate to produce distinctive changes in personality while others operate to select persons with distinctive characteristics to go on to the next stage.

The result of the process, extended over a considerable period of time, may be to produce distinctive personalities. By looking at both the social and the individual sources of such patterns we can better assess the extent to which entrants into an occupation begin with a set of distinctive characteristics that remain relatively unchanged, or the extent to which change is the result of particular factors in the process of training, entering and practicing the occupation.

Our guiding assumption is that personality characteristics are relevant for the analysis of an occupational role in two ways. First, the role may allow opportunities for the expression of certain personality characteristics. Second, the role, conceived of as a set of behaviors and attitudes which constitute a repertory, may be performed more easily by persons who possess particular personality characteristics.

It is the second perspective which characteristically guides the orientation of research on personality and occupational role. Applicants or entrants into an occupational role are examined to determine whether they possess a characteristic or typical personality profile. The process by which such a pattern may develop has not been explicated but it is possible that self-perception and self-selection can operate to produce distinctive patterns. For example, entrants perceive themselves as possessing those attitudes and traits that they believe to be "desired" or "expected" for persons entering the occupation. A process of self-selection then occurs and the degree of similarity between the personality needs of the entrants and the successful incumbents of the occupational role is largely affected by the extent to which entrants are accurate in their perception of their own characteristics and in their assessment of the requirements of the occupational role. If the selection is mediated by selecting agents such as school admission boards, then the expectations of these agents will also have to be considered.

An additional though not unrelated question is: How do these personality characteristics contribute to or facilitate the role performance of the person in the role? It cannot be assumed that role performance is automatically facilitated because there is a similarity, on a verbal level, between the definition of a particular personality need and the behavior or attitudes considered important for those who perform the role. For example, Nurturance as a need is defined on the EPPS as "to help friends when they are in trouble, to assist others, to do small favors for others, to be generous with others, to sympathize with others who are hurt or sick, to show a great deal of affection toward others, to have others confide in one about personal problems." The nursing role, on the face of it, would appear to involve behavior of the same kind; helping others, being generous to others and sympathizing with others. However, the appearance of congruity in the verbal description of the need and of the demands of the role does not mean that a person who has a high Nurturance need *performs* any better in the role of nurse than someone with a low Nurturance need. Determining the actual relation between personality characteristics and role performance is an empirical matter which cannot be assumed to be confirmed solely by the appearance of a high Nurturance need among a group of nurses as compared with non-nurses. Determining how personality characteristics contribute to or detract from effective role performance in particular occupations and institutional settings is difficult because clear criteria of successful performance of the role do not exist. The assessment of the relation between personality needs and effective role performance requires standards concerning "effectiveness." In addition, it must be noted that the behavioral correlates of personality needs have not been adequately determined.

We could not conclude, even if we were to discover a distinctive set of personality traits for nurses, that these traits contribute to their successful role performance. Essentially, what we are saying is that a correlation does not indicate a causal relationship. We could argue that the task of discovering the effect of personality characteristics on role performance requires first discovering the presence of a distinctive set of personality characteristics for incumbents of an occupational role. Certainly, the discovery of a pattern could then lead us to the exploration of how individuals demonstrating these traits actually function.

The approach we are taking is that of attempting to determine whether members of a particular occupational role, specifically nursing, are characterized by a distinctive set of personality needs. By drawing together several studies done at different times in various nursing schools which used the same instrument, we are able to examine the question more thoroughly than if we relied solely on our own data collected at one diploma school of nursing.

In addition, we are able to suggest a model for research that directs attention to the several stages in the process of becoming a member of an occupational role. Implications concerning the use of personality tests to select applicants to nursing schools also emerge from this analysis. At each stage of the model, it is possible and desirable to obtain data concerning the personality characteristics of those being socialized. The questions that can be posed and answered will vary at each stage but, viewed overall, such a model would enable us to orient research within a larger framework and gradually fit in those parts of the picture that are still unstudied.

STAGES IN OCCUPATIONAL ENTRY: A MODEL

1. Preference

Persons who are only considering an occupation and have not yet entered it or are not yet in training for it may be classified as having an expressed preference. Do those expressing a preference differ from those preferring other occupations? Do persons expressing preferences for different occupations differ in ways that would enable us to discriminate them from other groups of people?

2. Application for Training

Expressed preference turns into action at a later point in time. Application to enter an occupation may be a formal or informal process, depending on the training requirements. For some occupations there is no period of formal training or education which is separated from entry into the occupation itself, i.e., one learns while on the job. For others, the formal education may be a general educational experience which provides no explicit job-relevant training, e.g., a college education prior to selling real estate. For certain others, there is a pre-training general educational experience followed by explicit, formal training in job relevant skills, e.g., medicine and collegiate nursing programs. Still another pattern is that shown in hospital or diploma schools of nursing which provide training to a selected group of high-school graduates.

Applicants to a training program may differ from non-applicants. Presumably, self-selection is still the most important factor at this stage although encouragement by parents and friends or from high-school teachers and counselors can also operate to dissuade a person who otherwise would have selected himself (i.e., applied), from making application.

3. Selection for Training

At the selection stage, the applicants have been screened for admission into the training period. Accepted applicants may differ from those rejected by the selection agents and from non-applicants in systematic ways. It is conceivable that at this point a relatively homogeneous group is permitted to enter training and that later changes or influences are of lesser importance. This would be especially true if training programs adopted relatively uniform criteria for selecting applicants in terms of personality characteristics. Even if this were so, the characteristics which formed the basis of selection may change with maturation and development and what might start out as a homogeneous group could become heterogeneous over time. Therefore, it is important to compare those entering training with random samples of non-entrants in the population—preferably matched in terms of age, intelligence, socioeconomic level and any other relevant variables.

It must also be recognized that variations may exist in the selection procedures of different training institutions and, furthermore, the same institution may change its selection criteria over time. Therefore, it would be necessary to include more than one institution in any study and also sample the same institution at different times to determine the extent of variation within the same institution.

4. In-Training Stage

The group of students in training may be examined to determine how they differ from selected control groups such as non-nursing students of the same age. Students in each of the various years can be compared separately. The three years can also be combined to produce a sample of nursing students-in-training without regard to differences between year in school.

During the years in training, changes in the group of trainees may come from four general sources:

A. Age. Certain changes would be expected to occur due to maturation. These changes would be typical of persons of the same age-level who are not in training. Therefore, comparisons with relevant control groups would be necessary to determine the "effects" of age.

B. Training. The training program may influence or produce changes in personality. Presumably, the effects of the program would be to mold personality along those lines considered most desirable by socialization agents. Therefore, comparisons with groups of the same age undergoing a different type of training would be needed.

C. Role models. The successful trainee could come to resemble role models as represented by previous successful trainees in the same institution (becoming like other student nurses) or practicing nurses in the same hospital (becoming like staff nurses). Therefore, comparisons with groups of practicing nurses or more advanced students in the same institution would be needed.

D. Selective attrition. A weeding-out process whereby training agents select certain persons to continue the program can contribute to a more homogeneous group of graduates, particularly if the selection is made in terms of personality characteristics. In contrast, weeding out because of academic deficiencies may or may not have any relation to personality characteristics.

Self-selection can also contribute to increased homogeneity since trainees may choose to leave the program even though they are successfully meeting its standards and requirements. A variety of reasons may operate, however, some of which are more related to personality and occupational role considerations than others. For example, leaving because one cannot afford the costs of training is quite different from leaving because one has changed his interest or motivation to become a member of the occupation or because one marries and is unable to remain in the program (e.g., some diploma nursing programs do not allow students who marry to remain in training).

Those who leave may show, if they were followed and re-tested over a period of years, the same pattern of personality traits as those who remain and complete the program. The group of dropouts, and whatever subgroups might be classified within it, depending on reasons for leaving, would thus serve as a control group in assessing the effects of a training program on the group of initial applicants and trainees.

5. Professional Stage

At the completion of the training stage, all successful trainees have the choice of actually entering the occupation or not. Reasons for leaving may range from an inability to find employment, a change of mind or, particularly for women, marriage which may represent either a permanent or a temporary leave from the occupation. Of those who marry, some definitely expect to return to the occupation, whereas others are relatively certain that they will not again seek active work in the occupation. The more difficult and costly the training period, i.e., the greater the investment the student has in preparing for entry, the greater the likelihood that he will actively seek and eventually find work.[5]

At this point another set of selection procedures enters into the process. We have already referred to self-selection, but selection is also exercised by the agencies, institutions and professional associations that admit qualified trainees into the occupation. In the case of nursing, the graduate of the school must also pass her state licensing examination and then, because most nurses do not generally practice as independent professionals (except for private nurses contracting to work for private parties), seek employment with a hospital, agency, or institution. Each of these may introduce selection criteria so that a group of practicing nurses studied in any

---

[5] Psathas, G., Toward a Theory of Occupational Choice for Women, *Sociology and Social Research*, 52, 1968, pp. 253-268.

one setting represents those who have applied and been selected for employment.

A group of practicing nurses varying in years of working experience would include those who were retained by the institution (external selection) and had chosen to remain with the institution (self selection). Factors affecting retention and persistence would therefore be involved in producing a group of persons actively employed in the occupation.

Since such persons would be older than those in the training stage, relevant control groups would have to be selected to determine how these persons differed from persons of the same age and from persons employed in other occupations.

Subjects for studies such as those of Roe[6] are highly selected and successful members of an occupation. In essence, such persons represent a "distilled" sample of individuals for whom all selection procedures have operated. In contrast, a group of new entrants into an occupation has yet to experience some of the selection procedures which would have to be successfully completed before they become the successful, older elite of the profession.

The data collected in this study were combined with data available in the research literature to provide answers to some of the questions posed by the model. An outline of some of these findings is presented here with many of the details involved in the actual comparisons and statistical tests omitted. We wished to assess the state of our knowledge concerning the personality of student nurses and, therefore, in order to maintain comparability, we selected only those studies that used the same personality test, the Edwards Personal Preference Schedule. It is possible that the results obtained are not similar to those which would be found if other tests were used.

The Edwards Personal Preference Schedule (EPPS)[7] is a paper-pencil personality test which can be administered in group or individual testing. Statements constructed to represent the 15 needs being measured are presented in a series of paired comparisons. The respondent makes 225 choices and a score for each need is then calculated. Group means and standard deviations can be com-

---

[6] Roe, A., *The Psychology of Occupations, op. cit.*

[7] Edwards, A. L., *Edwards Personal Preference Schedule, Revised Manual,* Psychological Corp., New York, 1959.

puted for each need and group comparisons made using t-test for significance of the difference between means. P values, indicating the level of statistical significance, are given in the following tables. A p value of .05 should be read as meaning that the observed difference between groups compared would be expected to occur no more than 5 times out of 100. A description of each of the 15 needs follows.

Manifest Needs Associated with Each of the Edwards Personal Preference Schedule (EPPS) Variables

1. Ach Achievement: To do one's best, to be successful, to accomplish tasks requiring skill and effort, to be a recognized authority, to accomplish something of great significance, to do a difficult job well, to solve difficult problems and puzzles, to be able to do things better than others, to write a great novel or play.

2. Def Deference: To get suggestions from others, to find out what others think, to follow instructions and do what is expected, to praise others, to tell others that they have done a good job, to accept the leadership of others, to read about great men, to conform to custom and avoid the unconventional, to let others make decisions.

3. Ord Order: To have written work neat and organized, to make plans before starting on a difficult task, to have things organized, to keep things neat and orderly, to make advance plans when taking a trip, to organize details of work, to keep letters and files according to some system, to have meals organized and a definite time for eating, to have things arranged so that they run smoothly without change.

4. Exh Exhibition: To say witty and clever things, to tell amusing jokes and stories, to talk about personal adventures and experiences, to have others notice and comment upon one's appearance, to say things just to see what effect it will have on others, to talk about personal achievements, to be the center of attention, to use words that others do not know the meaning of, to ask questions others cannot answer.

5. Aut Autonomy: To be able to come and go as desired, to say what one thinks about things, to be independent of others in making decisions, to feel free to do what one wants, to do things that are unconventional, to avoid situations where one is expected to conform, to do things without regard to what others may think, to criticize those in positions of authority, to avoid responsibilities and obligations.

6. Aff Affiliation: To be loyal to friends, to participate in friendly groups, to do things for friends, to form new friendships, to make as many friends as possible, to share things with friends, to do things with friends rather than alone, to form strong attachments, to write letters to friends.

7. Int Intraception: To analyze one's motives and feelings, to observe others, to understand how others feel about problems, to put one's self in another's place, to judge people by why they do things rather than by what they do, to analyze the behavior of others, to analyze the motives of others, to predict how others will act.

8. Suc Succorance: To have others provide help when in trouble, to seek encouragement from others, to have others be kindly, to have others be sympathetic and understanding about personal problems, to receive a great deal of affection from others, to have others do favors cheerfully, to be helped by others when depressed, to have others feel sorry when one is sick, to have a fuss made over one when hurt.

9. Dom Dominance: To argue for one's point of view, to be a leader in groups to which one belongs, to be regarded by others as a leader, to be elected or appointed chairman of committees, to make group decisions, to settle arguments and disputes between others, to persuade and influence others to do what one wants, to supervise and direct the actions of others, to tell others how to do their jobs.

10. Aba Abasement: To feel guilty when one does something wrong, to accept blame when things do not go right, to feel that personal pain and misery suffered does more good than harm, to feel the need for punishment for wrong doing, to feel better when giving in and avoiding a fight than when having one's own way, to feel the need for confession of errors, to feel depressed by inability to handle situations, to feel timid in the presence of superiors, to feel inferior to others in most respects.

11. Nur Nurturance: To help friends when they are in trouble, to assist others less fortunate, to treat others with kindness and sympathy, to forgive others, to do small favors for others, to be generous with others, to sympathize with others who are hurt or sick, to show a great deal of affection toward others, to have others confide in one about personal problems.

12. Chg Change: To do new and different things, to travel to meet new people, to experience novelty and change in daily routine, to experiment and try new things, to eat in new and different places, to try new and different jobs, to move about the country and live in different places, to participate in new fads and fashions.

13. End Endurance: To keep at a job until it is finished, to complete any job undertaken, to work hard at a task, to keep at a puzzle or problem until it is solved, to work at a single job before taking on others, to stay up late working in order to get a job done, to put in long hours of work without distraction, to stick at a problem even though it may seem as if no progress is being made, to avoid being interrupted while at work.

14. Het Heterosexuality: To go out with members of the opposite sex, to engage in social activities with the opposite sex, to be in love with someone of the opposite sex, to kiss those of the opposite sex, to be regarded as physically attractive by those of the opposite sex, to participate in discussions about sex, to read books and plays involving sex, to listen to or to tell jokes involving sex, to become sexually excited.

15. Agg Aggression: To attack contrary points of view, to tell others what one thinks about them, to criticize others publicly, to make fun of others, to tell others off when disagreeing with them, to get revenge for insults, to become angry, to blame others when things go wrong, to read newspaper accounts of violence.

1. Preference

We have not located any studies nor does our own study include personality test data which would allow us to compare those who express a preference for nursing with those who express preferences for other occupations. Ideally, such data should be collected prospectively rather than retrospectively. That is, the preferences should be those expressed prior to the time of actual decision or application rather than asking persons who have already made their occupational "decisions" to think back to some earlier point in time and report what occupations they had "considered" or been "interested in." Following our model, such persons could be followed over time to determine how their preferences change and how their final decisions are related to their earlier expressed preferences.

2. Application for Training

Do high school seniors who apply to enter nursing school differ in their personality characteristics from those who do not apply?

Data are lacking which would enable us to answer this question. At this critical point in high school, it is possible that self-selection has the greatest effect although external influences such as encouragement or dissuasion by parents, relatives and high-school peers may also operate.

If differences exist, they may be the same differences, which, when found in later stages, are otherwise attributed to training effects. Early differences may be determinants of later differences or they may interact with other variables which, in turn, produce distinctive personality characteristics.

The testing of applicants to a particular school of nursing does not permit us to assess the selective effect of that particular school, whereas if we could obtain data from a sample of high-school girls it would also be possible to determine whether applicants to different schools of nursing differ from one another. Thus, the selective attracting effect of particular schools could also be assessed.

3. Selection for Training

Ideally, to answer the question of whether there are any personality traits specific to the group admitted for training, nursing students recently accepted for training should be compared with a group of applicants who were not admitted and with other immediate age peers. No data are available for unaccepted applicants. The only comparison possible is that between accepted applicants and a large sample of high-school girls representing a control group of age peers. Of the relevant data available, there are two studies[8, 9] in which accepted applicants were tested prior to or early in their

---

[8] Smith, G. M., The Role of Personality in Nursing Education, *Nursing Research, 14,* 1965, pp. 54–58, reported EPPS scores for high-school students who were successful applicants to the Catherine Laboure School of Nursing, a Roman Catholic 3-year diploma school of nursing, situated in the Greater Boston area. The girls, all of whom matriculated between 1957 and 1960, took the EPPS during their senior high-school year and were later admitted to the nursing school.

[9] Reece, M. M., Personality Characteristics and Success in a Nursing Program, *Nursing Research, 10,* 1961, pp. 172–176, reported scores for a group of 87 freshmen in a diploma school at Wayne State University. All were tested subsequent to the beginning of their training. Reece subdivided his group into 55 students who went on to successfully complete their nursing training and another 32 students who left school for various reasons (including academic failure, marriage, lack of interest) during the 3-year period.

freshman year. Smith tested accepted applicants during their senior year in high school. Of 264 applicants, 219 went on to successfully complete the program three years later, and 45 did not. The test scores of an additional 15 who left during the freshman year either to marry or for health or financial reasons were not reported. Because the girls had not been exposed to the possible influences of nursing training at the time of testing, they represent a group as yet uninfluenced by the school experience itself.

Reece reported scores of 87 freshmen tested early in their freshman year. Of these, 55 subsequently completed their nursing training and 32 did not.

In addition, test scores obtained from 79 freshmen at General Hospital, tested three months after the beginning of their freshman year in 1962, were available. Since these girls were followed for a period of three years, test scores are available for both the successful students and the dropouts.

Scores for a group of girls in high school, reported by Klett,[10] were available for comparison with these students.

How do high-school students who are later admitted to nursing school, but who when tested have not been exposed at all to nursing training, differ from a general sample of high-school girls?

The differences found between the 264 Catherine Laboure nursing school entrants reported by Smith and the 834 high-school girls in Klett's sample appear in Table 1. Unless those 15 students whose scores are missing from Smith's sample are so different from

---

[10] Klett, C. J., Performance of High School Students on the Edwards Personal Preference Schedule, *Journal of Consulting Psychology, 21,* 1957, pp. 68–72. This sample of EPPS scores was collected following administration of the test in two King County high schools outside the city of Seattle, Washington. One high school was located in an outlying town in the county, while the other was in an expanding residential suburban area of Seattle. Data were reported by Klett on a total of 834 high-school girls, of whom about 330 were sophomores, 280 juniors, and 200 seniors. No significant correlations were found between grades and need scores. Correlations between age and need scores were also very low (the highest being −.18) when a total group consisting of the 834 girls as well as 799 boys was considered. These low correlations make the use of the total group of high-school girls, rather than a group consisting only of seniors, justified in the comparisons reported in the present study.

Table 1

p value	Catherine Laboure Students Significantly Higher than High-School Girls		Catherine Laboure Students Significantly Lower than High-School Girls	
	.01 Level	.05 Level	.01 Level	.05 Level
	Def	None	Aut	None
	Int		Aff	
	Dom		Chg	
	Aba		Het	
	Nur		Agg	
	End			

the 264 students for whom data are reported as to change the pattern of differences reported above, we may conclude that, at least for the Catherine Laboure School of Nursing, the nursing student shows many personality differences from her peers even at a time prior to her entry into the nursing school. Either self selection or external selection may be involved in determining this pattern and probably a combination of both actually operated. Since only one school is involved in this comparison we hesitate to generalize about this pattern of differences.

How do freshman nursing students, tested after only a short period of nursing training, differ from a general sample of high-school girls?

Wayne State freshmen, of whom there were 87, were found to differ from high-school girls in the needs presented in Table 2.

Table 2

p value	Wayne State Students Significantly Higher than High-School Girls		Wayne State Students Significantly Lower than High-School Girls	
	.01 Level	.05 Level	.01 Level	.05 Level
	Int	Ach	Aut	None
	End		Aff	
			Suc	
			Agg	

The 79 General Hospital freshmen differed from high-school girls on the needs listed in Table 3.

Table 3

p value	General Hospital Students Significantly Higher than High-School Girls		General Hospital Students Significantly Lower than High-School Girls	
	.01 Level	.05 Level	.01 Level	.05 Level
	Int	Suc	**Ord**	**None**
		Nur	Agg	

Both the Wayne State and the General Hospital groups showed higher scores than the high-school group on Intraception and lower scores on Aggression. Other need scores were significantly different from the high-school group but not for both groups. On one need, Succorance, the direction of the significant difference between nursing student and high-school groups was opposite for each of the nursing student groups. Wayne State students were significantly lower than high-school girls on this need, General Hospital students were significantly higher.

When we consider the Catherine Laboure group, we note that there was agreement for all three groups on needs Intraception (higher than high-school girls) and Aggression (lower than high-school girls). This ageement occurred despite the fact that the Catherine Laboure group was tested at a slightly earlier age and prior to any possible training influence. It suggests that, at least for these two needs, certain personality characteristics typical of the nursing student may be present even before she enters nursing school. Thus, it is likely that they are due to factors operating *at this time,* rather than being formed as a result of training influences encountered after entry. This does not mean that these two needs, or any others, are not influenced during the period following the time of testing as a result of training or other experiences.

At this point in the analysis it appears that generalizations about the possession of certain personality characteristics, notably high Intraception and low Aggression, which extend beyond any one specific entering or freshman student group, are justified.

Despite some differences between the schools (Wayne State

freshmen were lower on Affiliation and Succorance and higher on Endurance than the General Hospital freshmen), these two samples were combined in order to produce a large group which could be considered representative of *freshmen* nursing students generally. We wanted to determine whether the same pattern of differences between nursing students and high-school students would remain and whether any other differences appeared. When Wayne State and General Hospital freshmen were combined to produce a single freshman group, they showed differences from high-school girls (Table 4). With the exception of the Achievement and Order

Table 4

	Freshman Nursing Students Significantly Higher than High-School Girls		Freshman Nursing Students Significantly Lower than High-School Girls	
p value	.01 Level	.05 Level	.01 Level	.05 Level
	Ach	None	Ord	None
	Int		Aut	
	Nur		Aff	
			Agg	

differences which did not previously show statistical significance, all of these differences were also found in the comparison of Catherine Laboure students with high-school girls.

In summary, it appears that freshmen nursing students are higher than a non-nursing control group of high-school girls on Intraception and Nurturance and lower on Autonomy, Affiliation and Aggression. Whether the same pattern will appear when comparisons are made between nursing students and older-age control groups remains to be determined. Thus far, we may generalize only for the admitted applicant and entering freshman group.

4. In-Training Stage

Before assessing changes that occur during the training stage, we wanted to compose a group of student nurses which would include first, second and third year students and determine whether any consistent differences existed in comparison with selected control groups.

In addition to the two freshman nursing-student groups already discussed, three other independent groups of students from diploma schools of nuring were available. These were 222 juniors in a diploma school in South Carolina,[11] 54 seniors at Barnes Hospital School of Nursing in St. Louis, to whom we administered the EPPS, and 53 seniors at General Hospital School of Nursing in a different class than the one reported previously.

In all, then, five independent nursing groups were available; two groups of freshmen, one group of juniors, and two groups of seniors.

These groups were combined to form one single "student nurse" group which could be compared with several comparison groups. Specifically, in addition to high-school girls, it was possible to make comparisons with college women,[12] adult women[13] and staff nurses.[14]

---

[11] Gynther, M. and Gertz, B., Personality Characteristics of Student Nurses in South Carolina, *Journal of Social Psychology, 56,* 1962, pp. 277-284.

[12] Edwards, A. L., *op. cit.,* reports EPPS scores for a group of 749 college women. The students were enrolled in day or evening liberal arts classes at various universities and though not stated by Edwards, it can probably be assumed that the subjects had been drawn from a number of different age levels.

[13] Edwards, A. L., *op. cit.,* also reports norms for a group of adult women comprised of 4,932 female household heads from urban and rural areas of 1,181 counties in 48 states, all of whom were members of a consumer purchase panel used for market surveys.

[14] Williamson, H. M., Edmonston, W. E., and Stern, J. A., Use of the EPPS for Identifying Personal Role Attributes Desirable in Nursing, *Journal of Health and Human Behavior, 4,* 1963, pp. 266–275. The staff-nurse group was composed of three groups. One, consisting of 32 nurses from a St. Louis general hospital, was reported by Williamson, Edmonston and Stern. The second group was made up of 50 nurses from another St. Louis hospital tested in the course of our research and the third was a group of 167 general medical and surgical nurses reported by Navran, L. and Stauffacher, J. C., A Comparative Analysis of the Personality Structure of Psychiatric and Nonpsychiatric Nurses, *Nursing Research, 7,* 1958, pp. 64-67. The three groups were combined into a single staff-nurse group, $N = 249$, despite the fact that there were differences among them.

A. Age. The college women were similar to nursing students in terms of age and continued involvement in the educational process, but differed in terms of higher socioeconomic status and measured intelligence. To the extent that EPPS need scores are related to socioeconomic status and intelligence, the comparisons of the two groups would be affected. The sample of adult women represented a cross-section of the U. S. population unbiased in terms of socioeconomic status or level of measured intelligence.

Comparisons between the "student-nurse" group and each of the comparison groups are summarized in Tables 5 and 6. Only those needs which showed statistically significant differences for three or more comparisons are shown in Table 5 and those showing differences for two comparisons in Table 6.

Table 5. EPPS Needs which Show Significant Differences between Student Nurses (N = 495) and at least Three Comparison Groups

	Comparison Groups			
	High School	College Women	Adult Women	Staff Nurses
Student Nurses higher than	Het	Het	Het	Het
		Nur	Nur	Nur
Student Nurses lower than		Ach	Ach	Ach
		Def	Def	Def
	Aut	Aut	Aut	
	Aff	Aff	Aff	

Student nurses were consistently higher on need Heterosexuality in all four comparisons. They were also higher on need Nurturance than three of the comparison groups and, it will be recalled, freshman nurses also tended to score higher than high-school girls.

Student nurses were lower on need Achievement, Deference, Autonomy and Affiliation in three comparisons. Intraception showed a consistent pattern only in two comparisons while differences on Abasement were not consistent.

Considerable support is found in these results for describing the personality of the "student nurse" as high on needs Hetero-

Table 6. EPPS Needs which Show Significant Differences between Student
          Nurses (N = 495) and at least Two Comparison Groups

| | Comparison Groups | | | |
	High School	College Women	Adult Women	Staff Nurses
Student Nurses higher than	Int	Aba[a]	Int	Aba[a]
Student Nurses lower than	Aba[a]			

[a] Inconsistent pattern

sexuality and Nurturance and low on needs Autonomy, Affiliation,
Achievement and Deference.

B. Training. These results do not reveal the manner in which
changes in personality needs were occurring nor the sources of such
changes. For example, by adding together all student nurses we
cannot indicate whether need Heterosexuality increased with each
year in school either longitudinally or cross-sectionally. Nor is it
clear whether any increase or decrease could be attributed to the
effects of training, selective attrition, or maturation. A more detailed breakdown of the nursing groups and comparisons with the
comparison groups is indicated.

A series of such comparisons was performed using as the framework for the analysis a design proposed by Campbell and Stanley.[15]

---

[15] Campbell, D. T. and Stanley, J. C., "Experimental and Quasi-
Experimental Designs for Research on Teaching," Chapter 5 in
Gage, N. L. (ed.), *Handbook of Research on Teaching,* Rand Mc-
Nally, Chicago, 1963, p. 230. They note that a "combination of longitudinal and cross-sectional comparisons should be more systematically
employed in developmental studies. The cross-sectional study by
itself confounds maturation with selection and mortality. The longitudinal study confounds maturation with repeated testing and with
history. It alone is probably better than the cross-sectional though
its greater cost gives it higher prestige. The combination, perhaps
with repeated cross-sectional comparisons at various times, seems
ideal."

The design involves employing cross-sectional and longudinal, as well as general population comparison groups to study the effects of a common variable, such as training. The specific details of this analysis have been reported elsewhere[16] and only an overview of the results is presented here.

The logic of the design enables us to clarify the extent to which changes in EPPS need scores were a result of training, selective attrition, or maturation. All students at the General Hospital School of Nursing, including those who dropped out and were later contacted, completed the EPPS twice.

The results show that for two needs, Deference and Heterosexuality, training clearly was associated with higher scores. Order and Aggression also showed increases, whereas Endurance and Intraception decreased. For these latter four needs, the effects of training were not as clear or consistent.

There were expected maturational effects which training appeared to attenuate in the case of Achievement, Dominance and Change and to enhance in the case of Autonomy. An attenuated effect means that student nurses change in the same direction as relevant age groups but not to the same extent. Enhancing effects indicate a change that is greater than expected.

On three needs, Affiliation, Abasement and Nurturance, maturation effects operated since all groups changed in the same direction as relevant age groups.

For two remaining needs, Succorance and Exhibition, no consistent pattern appeared.

On the basis of this analysis, it is possible to say that training affects certain personality needs by changing, attenuating or enhancing normal, expected maturational changes. Other needs appear to remain unaffected by the nursing training experience.

C. Role models. Another comparison of nursing students involved determining whether they become more similar to or different from role models represented by previous generations of students at the same school (e.g., another senior class) or staff nurses employed at the hospital in which the school is located.

These comparisons were made and it was found that successful students did not become more similar to seniors at the same school

---

[16] Psathas, G. and Plapp, J., Assessing the Effects of Training: A Problem in Design, *Nursing Research,* 1968, in press.

(class of 1963). Freshmen differed significantly from seniors on four needs (Deference, Exhibition, Intraception, higher for freshmen, Heterosexuality, lower for freshmen) and when these same freshmen were tested in their senior year, they differed from the senior sample on five needs (Exhibition, Autonomy and Aggression, higher; Affiliation and Abasement, lower) only one of which was the same as when they were observed as freshmen. If they were becoming more similar to the seniors, fewer differences would be expected in the senior-senior comparison than in the freshman-senior comparison.

Compared with the same senior sample, the dropouts, considered as a group, showed greater similarity to the successful seniors when the dropouts were tested three years after they entered school. There were differences on five needs at the time of first testing (Deference, Affiliation, Nurturance, higher for the dropout group; Heterosexuality and Aggression lower) compared with no significant differences at the time of second testing. This unexpected finding emphasizes the fact that we are not justified in stating that successful students become more like previous seniors in the same school. In fact, three years after entering school, the dropouts were more similar to previous seniors than were the successful students.

Secondly, there was also little evidence for the view that student nurses become like staff nurses. There were about the same number of differences between the EPPS scores of the seniors and the staff nurses as there were between the freshmen and the staff nurses. In their freshman year, successful students differed from the staff nurses on seven needs: they were higher than staff nurses on Exhibition, Intraception, Succorance, Abasement and Nurturance, and lower on Order and Endurance. By the time they themselves were seniors they differed from the staff nurses on six needs, with only two of the same needs showing differences. At a time when we would expect them to be more similar to the staff nurses, they were higher than staff nurses on Exhibition, Autonomy, Heterosexuality and Aggression, and lower on Deference and Endurance.

Therefore, the nursing student, as judged by results from this one school of nursing, does not become more like those who may be role models for her, i.e., seniors or staff nurses. It is also noteworthy that successive classes of graduating seniors from the same school differed. This would indicate that the environmental "press" either did not operate in a consistent fashion, or that successive entering classes were sufficiently different so that the interaction effect of initial differences plus training effects resulted in variable "products" in succeeding years. Detailed study of successive generations of students in the same school is needed to assess the effect of that school's training on the personality of the student nurse.

D. *Selective attrition.* In order to assess the effect of selective attrition on these comparisons, we wished to determine whether those students who left school differed in any systematic way from those who successfully completed the program. Because the testing of these students occurred at the time of entry, we felt that this comparison would be relevant in determining whether success in school can be predicted on the basis of EPPS needs.

Looking first at General Hospital successful students, they were found to be higher than the unsuccessful ones on one need, Intraception; this is also one of the five needs that characterized the entering student nurse when compared with the high-school control group.

Looking at other schools, the Catherine Laboure successful students, compared with those who left by the end of their *first* year, showed that the successful students were higher on Achievement and lower on Heterosexuality. In Reece's study, dropouts at any time within the *three* years were compared with successful students. The successful students were lower on Achievement and higher on Deference.

Thus, on only one need, Achievement, were significant differences found in more than one school, but the directions are opposite. The other needs which differentiate between successful and unsuccessful students were not consistent from one school to another.

Differences in the studies may account for the findings since Smith tested students while they were still seniors in high school, whereas subjects in our study and that by Reece were tested after they entered nursing school. Smith examined only the first-year dropout group, whereas Reece included the dropouts from all three years. But even though Reece's study and the General Hospital study are comparable in this regard, no consistent pattern was found. Further, even when we compared only the General Hospital *first-year* dropouts with the successful students, as Smith did, no significant differences on any EPPS need were found.

These results suggest that no EPPS need or pattern of needs

consistently predicts across schools to successful completion of either the first or the entire three years of nursing school.

Within the dropout group there were differences in terms of time of leaving and stated reason for leaving school. It is conceivable that some consistent pattern of EPPS needs differentiates subgroups of students within the general dropout category.

For example, those who fail for academic reasons may represent a group that differs more from the successful students than those who leave to marry. The latter group may represent persons who are still interested in becoming nurses but who, when confronted with an opportunity to marry, choose to do so and leave. The first group would represent the kind of student the school is most interested in screening out, whereas the latter may be regarded as an undesirable loss to nursing.

With regard to time of leaving school, some students may have greatest difficulty with new situations and are unsuccessful in persisting past the first year. Others may have difficulty only as they move closer to the completion of the program. There is a relation between time of leaving and reason for leaving, however, since academic failures tend to occur more often in the freshman year, whereas marriages occur more frequently after the first year. Nevertheless, both comparisons are included here.

When we compared successful General Hospital students with 17 of their peers who dropped out of school during their freshman year we found that there were no significant differences between these two groups on any EPPS need. Similarly, no significant differences were found between the freshman EPPS scores of the 49 successful students and the 13 of their peers who dropped out of schools after their freshman year. There were also no significant differences between the freshman EPPS scores of these two dropout groups, i.e., first-year and later dropouts did not show significant differences from one another.

Time of leaving school was not associated with any pattern of EPPS needs and therefore personality, as measured by this test, does not seem to be an important predictor of successful school completion.

A different subdivision of the dropout group was made in terms of "reasons for leaving school" as classified in the school's official records. The freshman EPPS scores of the 49 successful students were compared with the freshman EPPS scores of those who were

officially classified as leaving because of dislike of nursing school
(N = 10), failure (N = 12), and marriage (N = 8). When the
dropout group was subdivided in this way, a number of significant differences appeared. Successful students were not significantly different from those students who left school because of
failure. However, successful students were significantly higher in
Intraception than those who left school because they disliked
nursing. This is one need on which entering nursing students
had been found to be significantly higher than high-school girls.
Finally, successful students were significantly higher in Aggression
and lower in Dominance than students who left school in order
to marry.

Although there is some variation within the total group of
dropouts when reason for leaving school is considered, there is not
sufficient evidence in these comparisons to warrant any conclusion
that there are distinct subgroups of dropouts characterized by distinctive sets of personality traits. In Chapter 3 a more detailed
discussion of the classification of dropouts offers additional reasons
for expecting few differences between themselves and successful
students.

5. Professional Stage

Staff nurses, currently employed in hospitals, represent one group
of successful trainees who have entered and remained in the occupation. Selective factors have already operated to lead some graduates
into other occupations, into temporary or permanent withdrawal
from nursing because of marriage, or into other settings in which
they may work as nurses. Personality differences may exist between
nurses who choose different specialties in the hospital (e.g., psychiatric, surgical and general duty nurses) and between nurses who
choose employment in different settings (e.g., hospital, private duty,
office, industry, school). We chose to compare staff nurses employed
in two local hospitals with normative comparison groups. These
staff nurses may be regarded as representing a varied group in
terms of age, years of experience and schools in which they were
trained. We believed that by grouping them together and comparing them with high-school girls, college women, adult women and
nursing-school students, we could assess the extent to which consistent differences or patterns of differences on personality needs
may exist.

Staff nurses were found to be low in Nurturance, Affiliation and Succorance when compared with each of the four other groups. They were also lower in Autonomy than all of the comparison groups except nursing students. On Abasement they were lower than all of the comparison groups except college women.

Remaining differences between staff nurse and other groups were more difficult to interpret, since there were inconsistencies in the directions of the differences. For example, while staff nurses were significantly *lower* than college women, high-school girls and nursing students on Exhibition and Heterosexuality, they were also significantly *higher* than adult women on each of these needs. Similarly, while staff nurses were significantly higher than these same three comparison groups on Deference, Order, and Endurance, they were significantly lower than adult women on these needs. Nevertheless, keeping these qualifications in mind, the staff nurse may be described as low in Exhibition and Heterosexuality and high in Deference, Order, and Endurance, except in comparison with adult women. On two other needs, Autonomy and Abasement, they were lower than adult women, but not significantly so, for one of the other three comparison groups. In order to interpret these results as showing the lasting effects of nursing training and nursing per se on personality, we made one additional comparison.

We examined all needs for which *both* staff nurses and the "student-nurse" group described earlier differed significantly and in the same direction when compared with the various normative groups.

Student and staff-nurse groups both obtained significantly higher scores than high-school girls on need Endurance, and significantly lower scores than high-school girls on needs Autonomy, Affiliation, Abasement, Exhibition and Change. Both nursing groups were significantly lower than college women on needs Autonomy, Affiliation and Dominance. Compared with adult women they were significantly higher on needs Heterosexuality, Exhibition, Intraception and Dominance, and significantly lower on needs Achievement. Deference, Autonomy, Affiliation, Order and Endurance. The only needs which were significantly in the same direction in each comparison were Autonomy and Affiliation, both being low for student and staff nurses. In terms of the present set of data, these two needs may be interpreted as reflecting personality differences between nurses and other women that persist over time.

CONCLUSION

Despite the gaps in data which the design we have outlined requires for the assessment of the distinctive personality characteristics of the student nurse, several patterns have emerged from the data available.

The most frequent and stable finding for groups of entering students is that they are relatively high on need Intraception and relatively low on need Aggression. In addition, other comparisons show that they are high on Nurturance and low on Autonomy and Affiliation.

This combination indicates a need to help others, give assistance, be generous, etc. (Nur), combined with a strong interest in analyzing, observing and understanding others (Int). This outgoing yet introspective interest in others is combined with the desire to be of assistance and service to them.

Their low interest in asserting independence, and achieving freedom from convention and supervision (Aut) can be adaptive in the school and hospital situation which puts them in a subordinate position with little independence or freedom from supervision and where judgments concerning their proper and conforming behavior are continually made. Similarly, being unassertive, not argumentative and critical of others, not vengeful or easy to anger can serve the student to advantage.

Their low scores on Affiliation indicate less loyalty to friends, less ease in developing intimate relationships and friendships, and less desire to form strong attachments to particular others. This resembles a "distance-keeping" mechanism which, combined with the other needs described above, represents a pattern of interest in helping others but not getting too close or, stated slightly differently, a desire to analyze, observe and understand others but not to become too involved with them. A low interest in being assertive and independent fits with the high Nurturance and Intraception pattern to characterize the entering student as one who is willing to accept rules, established procedures and orders, and is more interested in helping and understanding others.

When large numbers of students in all years in school are compared with non-nursing controls and with staff nurses, student nurses appear to "lose" their interest in understanding others (Intraception is not significant) and "develop" an interest in heterosexual activities which can be interpreted as turning toward more effective relationships with the opposite sex. This is quite different from the initially high Nurturance need of entering students which indicated an interest in activities generally regarded as more relevant in their dealings with patients.

The senior students are still low on Autonomy and Affiliation and they are now also low on Achievement and Deference. A lower Achievement need score represents a decline in interest to do well, to be successful and accomplish something or to overcome obstacles. They become less interested in following instructions, praising others, doing what is expected, accepting leadership and conforming to custom (Def). In short, they appear to have more casual interests in performing well in those behaviors that are most relevant to conforming to hospital and school routines or excelling in the performance of duties. They are less deferent but they do show increases in Autonomy. However, Aggression is no longer significantly low so they are moving, to some extent, in the direction of greater assertiveness.

In assessing the effects of training on the changes in personality needs, it was found that for the General Hospital school group most specifically, training is associated with an increase in Heterosexuality and a decrease in Deference. Order and Aggression also increase with training but Endurance and Intraception decline.[17] Thus, the decline in interest in analyzing, observing and understanding others is one effect of training that operates on a clearly established distinctive trait of entering freshmen. An interest in order, planning, neatness and maintenance of smoothly functioning arrangements (Ord) develops and, needless to say, this represents a functionally significant aspect of performance in the nursing role.

---

[17] Levitt, E. E., Lubin, B., and Zuckerman, M., The Student Nurse, the College Woman and the Graduate Nurse: A Comparative Study, *Nursing Research, 11,* 1962, pp. 80-82, using student nurses in a collegiate program, also noted a decrease in needs Nurturance and Endurance, a higher score on Heterosexuality than adult women, and increases in Order. However, Deference increases. They conclude that "by the time she has practiced for some years, the student's goals had shifted from the need to serve suffering humanity—which was probably her main reason for choosing nursing as a career—to attention to technical skills, routine and ritual, and to supervisors and doctors as the major source of approval."

As Aggression increases (and as the change in Autonomy is enhanced by training) it appears that the student nurses are moving in the direction of greater independence, assertiveness and expression of negative affect. However, training attenuates an expected age-related increase in Dominance, i.e., the need to lead others, achieve leadership positions, persuade and influence others and supervise and direct the activities of others. Thus, the assertion and independence that develop seem to be more intra-personally oriented in the sense of wanting to be free of others, rather than reflecting a need to influence and control others. The interpersonal focus in need Aggression represents a critical and argumentative stance rather than the assumption of responsibility.

The decline in need Endurance and the lack of an expected age-related increase in need Achievement indicate that needs which are most directly related to keeping at a job—persistence in working hard and putting in long hours—do not increase in strength. Given the nature of nursing, such orientations would be relevant to and functional for the performance of nursing duties. That is, nursing demands effort and energy, attention to detail and the observance of routine. The concern for order, detail and neatness (Ord) represents an investment in the ritualized performance of tasks rather than interest in accomplishing and achieving goals, or deriving satisfaction from the application of effort and energy (Ach).

In addition, training attenuates expected age-related increases in need Change. This pattern supports the notion that novelty, experimentation and change of routine and behavior become less important while interest in successful goal-attainment also declines.

The comparison of those who leave with those who successfully complete the training program shows that no significant pattern of needs characterizes those who leave when these are considered as a group. Only for subgroups of dropouts, such as those who leave because of dislike of nursing (successful students are higher on Intraception) and those who leave to marry (successful students are higher in Aggression and lower on Dominance) do significant differences appear. These differences show that one need that characterized entering students, Intraception, is related importantly to success for some students. Too low an Aggression need and too high a Dominance need are, for some students, either hindrances in their successful completion of training or functional to their achieving marriage earlier than their peers. Interestingly enough, those who marry are not significantly different on need Heterosexuality.

The pattern of "becoming" like role models such as staff nurses or seniors is not found for nursing students. The graduating seniors show more differences than similarities to these significant others. For the "model" groups there are a number of sources of variation that could not be controlled in the comparisons made and we cannot conclude that "successful" students, compared with more carefully selected model groups, would not show different patterns. However, we did expect that one "generation" (i.e., class) of students in the same school would become more similar to a preceding class in that school but, in contrast, those who dropped out of school showed fewer differences from the comparison group than those who completed the program and became seniors themselves.

The results of a study by Williamson, Edmonston and Stern[18] are relevant in evaluating whether the changes we have noted as occurring for the student nurse are in a "desirable" direction. They asked administrative nursing staff at a St. Louis general hospital to rank the EPPS traits according to whether they felt the trait was desirable in the ideal staff nurse. The results of the rankings showed that the highest five EPPS needs were Achievement, Order, Intraception, Deference and Affiliation. The five needs which received the lowest ranks were Autonomy, Succorance, Heterosexuality, Exhibition and Aggression.

The results of the present study show that changes occur in the course of nursing training in a direction which is not considered "desirable" by nursing staff. Specifically, although at the time of entry into school, Intraception, one of the five desirable needs, is high, and Autonomy and Aggression, two of the least desirable, are low, at the time of graduation scores in Autonomy and Aggression have increased and Achievement and Deference have declined. In addition, Succorance and Heterosexuality rise rather than decline and Deference and Affiliation decline rather than rise. If anything, then, changes in the student nurse are occurring in a direction opposite to that which would be considered desirable by a group of judges such as administrative nursing staff.

What is the nursing student like in terms of personality needs?

---

18 Williamson, H. M., Edmonston, W. E., and Stern, J. A., Use of the EPPS for Identifying Personal Role Attributed Desirable in Nursing, *Journal of Health and Human Behavior, 4,* 1963, pp. 266-275.

In summary, she is likely, at the time of entry into nursing school, to be high on needs Intraception and Nurturance and low on Aggression and Autonomy.

The school experience is associated with an increase in needs Heterosexuality, Order and Aggression. An expected age-related increase in need Autonomy is enhanced by training. A decline appears in needs Deference, Endurance and Intraception. Training attenuates an expected age-related increase in Dominance, Achievement and Change.

The general pattern that emerges is one of a person who does not seek power and control over others but at the same time is becoming critical, resentful and less willing to be dependent on or deferent to others. She is not motivated to achieve success or gain satisfaction via the investment of self and energy in work nor is there a willingness to change, experiment or modify the life situation. She also becomes less motivated by a need to help and serve others (Nurturance shows a general maturational increase) or to observe, understand, and analyze others or herself. One major change that occurs in the student nurse is manifested by a striking rise in interest in the expression of and satisfaction of heterosexual needs.

The changes and effects noted do not provide a favorable picture of an "ideal" nurse who is motivated to serve, derives satisfaction from alleviating suffering and accepts her role as "ministering angel." These girls are not Florence Nightingales nor is it reasonable to expect that they would become replicas of her. On the other hand, they are not developing in the direction of "leaders of the profession." They are not interested in achieving positions of prominence, effecting change, or asserting themselves. Although there is some evidence of a dissatisfaction with subordinate status, this tends to be a more passive adaptation than an active, change-oriented stance.

Acceptance of the status quo may be what is reflected in the increasing scores on need Order while at the same time there is an expression of an interest in "escape," if we can so interpret the rise of need Heterosexuality. Sex, dating and marriage become dominant interests. Scores on this need decline for staff nurses but, even so, their scores remained higher than those for adult women on this need.

What the long-term changes will be for student nurses after leaving school and entering the world of work, in which changes are currently occurring, cannot be stated at this time. The prediction we would venture is that the leadership sought by the nursing profession is not likely to come from the typical diploma school graduate. And of even more significance we feel, is the fact that the pattern of personality needs shown by the successful student is not consistent with the "ideal" role performance of the nurse *qua* nurse, i.e., as one seeking self-fulfillment through service to others.

Chapter 6

Small Schools, Rules and Evaluations*

Students in small schools are often confronted with problems which are technically unrelated to the formal socialization goals of the institution. Behind the "kid-glove" treatment which many small schools engage in, lies the tendency for "total person evaluation" which often proves stifling and frustrating for students who fail to conform. The "home away from home" character of small schools may be intolerable for students who wish to establish or to maintain some measure of autonomy. Student officers often function as cadres for school administrations. The system possesses attributes which press toward encroachment upon student privacy. Subjective, "personalized" evaluation by administrators may be as punitive to some students as it is charitable to others. From one theoretical perspective, the "goody-goods" are as deviant as the "wild ones." Specific structural changes in small school systems might increase the correlation between ability and receiving a degree.

---

* This chapter was written by Cynthia Krueger, formerly at the Center of Community and Metropolitan Studies, University of Missouri at St. Louis, and now at the Department of Sociology-Anthropology, Brooklyn College.

SMALL SCHOOLS, RULES AND REGULATIONS:
AN ARGUMENT FOR REFORM

Small institutions—colleges as well as nursing schools—often pose unnecessary difficulties for their students. Some of these difficulties also exist in large institutions; indeed, they are inherent in the socialization process. Others emerge primarily because the institution is small. In this chapter we shall be concerned with institutions in which "kid gloves" and "personalized" treatment, rather than "red tape," place hurdles in the student's path.

There are nursing school situations in which the ability of certain students to operate within the school rules and regulations is more problematic, with respect to successful completion of the program, than is their talent or intelligence. Few school administrators would admit to the existence of such situations, but the fact that they do exist is evident in the various warning and probation systems, counseling programs, and arrangements for consultations with parents that schools engage in as part of a complicated effort to retain their focus on training or education. (It should be noted that the more direct question of whether or not the rules themselves should be changed, or even eliminated, is customarily the last alternative considered and most seldom chosen.) The sets of rules within which students live includes both specific "do's" and "don'ts" and sweeping admonitions for the students to display "correct" or "proper" behavior. Only some of the rules are technically related to the formal socialization goals of the institution, and only some of them exist *outside* the institution; many of the regulations are peripheral to these goals, and exist only *within* the school, i.e., they are "institutionally specific." Although the relevance of the goal-peripheral rules is sometimes questioned by students, school administrators often treat them with utmost seriousness.

RULE RECALCITRANCE

Some rules are championed by administrators because they are "part of our tradition." Other rules appear to have emerged with the laying of the cornerstone of the students' dormitory. A most durable class of rules appears to exist to placate parents. Many schools pride themselves on their parent-like attitudes—attitudes which sometimes cause the students to feel that the schools are out-parenting the parents. The conflicts which such a relationship breeds are difficult to resolve because the confrontation occurs precisely at a time when students wish to express their independence and, indeed, in many other areas of their experience they are being encouraged to become independent. It is most frustrating, therefore, for the student to be confronted with a kind of institutional super-parent, often more rigid and demanding than the parents whom the student has, in a sense, left behind. The *in loco parentis* rule constitutes a principle employed explicitly in some schools and implicitly in others but, in our society, it is particularly and almost invariably applied to female students in colleges and other educational institutions. Activation of this principle may be viewed as a special application of the more general societal procedures for maintaining female virtue because, given the present attitudes toward female behavior, institutions which are dedicated to the training of females generally have what amounts to a tacit agreement with parents to function as bastions of their daughters' morality. Consequently, such institutions operate in a structural environment which encourages them to occupy a custodial status with regard to their students' private lives, regardless of the effort required and the possible deleterious effects on the students.

Despite the principle of *in loco parentis* which is sold to parents, the schools customarily are required (or find it expedient) to use a legalistic approach to justify their actions and their expressions of what they expect of students. Given that schools feel a responsibility to control the private lives of the students, some mechanism for operationalizing that aim must be devised. The school's behavioral "territory," i.e., the range of behavior it can hope to control, must be staked out in advance; generally, this is accomplished through a network of school rules. The reliance of administrators upon rules to justify their actions means that rules form the basis of their authority, and this contributes to the press which they feel to "make the rules stick." Additional rules are often required to eliminate all loopholes which the students might find and use in interpreting the basic rules. The closer the school guards its authority over the students the more ancillary rules are required, and the greater is the students' feeling of being hemmed in by a system constructed of petty bureaucratic restrictions with some administrator pulling the strings.[1]

---

[1] Gouldner, Alvin W., in *Patterns of Industrial Bureaucracy*, The Free Press, Glencoe, Illinois, 1954, p. 178, discusses a similar process in

It is obvious that institutions such as nursing schools have a vested interest in keeping to a minimum all factors which might conceivably interfere with students' successful completion of the school program. The crucial point, however, is the determination of precisely which factors should be designated as disruptive of goal-attainment. Often the school and the students disagree on this point. Nonetheless, the institution's output is its graduates, and those who fail—or who are perceived as contributing to the failure of others—constitute an institutional deficit, a bad investment. In addition, because the behavior of the graduates of an institution is believed to affect the reputation of the school, the organization often maintains a form of "quality control" over the character as well as over the expertise of the individuals to whom it expects to award diplomas. Regardless of how numerous they may be, specific rules and technical requirements governing students are occasionally perceived by administrators to be inadequate for this task; hence, mandates requiring "proper" conduct and the "right attitude" are often employed by the school to supplement other weeding-out mechanisms. From the point of view of the students, a rule such as one requiring "proper conduct" may operate to destroy all loopholes yet remaining in the set of established regulations, as well as to cover situations not anticipated by these regulations.

TOTAL PERSON EVALUATION: MANDATES AND CADRES

For most school administrators, the body of rules provides a framework within which students are evaluated. From an administrative

---

the industrial setting. He states: "To put it more sharply, bureaucratic rules seem to be sustained not only because they mitigate some tensions, but also, because they *preserve* and allow other *tensions* to persist. If bureaucratic rules are a 'defense mechanism,' they not only defend the organization from certain tensions (those coming from close supervision) but they also *defend other tensions* as well (those conducing the close supervision) ." Thus, bureaucratic rules are often a poor substitute for an effective social control system; if the rules solved the problems to which they address themselves, they would assure their own dissolution. In the school setting, establishing a rule prohibiting an action does not eradicate the conditions leading to students' engaging in that action, much less the conditions leading to the school's prohibiting it.

point of view, conformity to rules indicates underlying attributes of "respect for authority," cooperativeness, consideration for others and the ability to abide by rules—in itself a mark of maturity. This interpretation of the school rules as being bench marks of the requisites of society renders the rules themselves symbolic of that which is socially sanctified. The sanctity of rules ultimately enables administrators to evaluate students who conform to rules as being of "good" moral character and, conversely, to evaluate those who deviate as being of questionable moral certification. The importance of even the most innocuous rule thus becomes magnified because of its symbolic moral nature, and one's reactions to rules becomes symptomatic of his "total person." Goffman[2] has noted: "Built right into the social arrangements of an organization, then, is a thoroughly embracing conception of the member—and not merely a conception of him *qua* member, but behind this a conception of him *qua* human being." It is through the establishment of rules that the conception of a student *qua* human being is applied to individuals. Students' reactions to the rules of a school are a vital means by which they give evidence that they either do or do not "fit" that total person conception. And, for the organization to activate its conception of a total human being, characteristics common to a "total institution" are developed.

On the latter topic, Goffman[3] has observed: "The central feature of total institutions can be described as a breakdown of the barriers ordinarily separating these three spheres of life (sleep, play and work)." Although Goffman's subsequent discussion deals with structural aspects of a total institution, his description of the entrapment of individuals most often resolves into the fact of centralized evaluation for all spheres of an individual's life. Thus, control of students by the institution results not only from the absolute number of rules in force; it is also a product of the inextricable blending of quite different normative orders—those governing standards of propriety and gratification and those governing expertise.[4] The most

---

[2] Goffman, Erving, *Asylums: Essays on the Social Situation of Mental Patients and Other Inmates,* Anchor Books, Doubleday and Company, Inc., Garden City, 1961, p. 180.

[3] *Ibid.,* p. 6.

[4] Gouldner and Gouldner discuss the *"standard of gratificational adequacy,* in which we appraise people and their behavior in terms of the enjoyment with which they provide us or the sheer amount

telling effect of this normative blend is that failure in one normative order may threaten the student's chances of success in the other. Not only may a student be expelled from school for other than academic reasons but the tolerance for borderline academic performance is often significantly affected by the student's extracurricular record. Reports of small-school administrators' attempts to "guide" new faculty members' grading policies, for example, are legion.

A second factor which adds to the total institution character of a school is the *interaction* between such institutional mandates as those calling for "the right attitude" and "proper conduct" and the body of objective rules. The plethora of rules and regulations virtually assures that few, if any, individuals will be able to exist within the institution without at some time or other breaking at least some of them. Thus, the rules establish universalistic guilt, and the vulnerability many students feel toward punishment reflects a realistic appraisal of their situation. On the other hand, students are informed that punishment for rule infractions will be geared to the individual case, i.e., it is particularistic. The content of punishment imposed in an individual case, however, is decided by administrators; thus, a student can never be certain that charity will be dispensed in regard to his particular transgression. As a general rule of thumb, then, guilt is established by the rules but punishment is often determined by whether or not the administrator views the student as having the "right attitude."

Any discussion of social control in a school setting would be incomplete without acknowledging the existence of "student governments." Although the character of student government varies somewhat from school to school, student government associations most often are identified as being "rubber stamps" for the administration. Student government leaders frequently associate with administrators on various boards or in consultation, where they are exposed at close range to problems encountered by the administration in running the school. This customarily results in effective socializa-

---

of gratification that we experience from them. On the other hand, there is the *standard of moral propriety* in which we appraise things, people, or actions in terms of the degree to which they conform with our conceptions of the way they ought to or should be." Gouldner, Alvin W. and Gouldner, Helen P., *Modern Sociology*, Harcourt, Brace and World, Inc., New York, 1963, pp. 569-572.

tion of cadres destined to link the administration's wishes into the mechanism established for student "expression." Above all, student officers function as role models of institutionally defined success to which all other students should aspire. In return, they are labelled as being leaders (a quality which, although seldom examined, is worshipped in our society) and often share in the making of minor decisions, though seldom in the determination of their content. The zeal with which student officers approach their positions of authority is notorious; often administrators are aghast at the sanctions the cadres would apply to their peers, and privately express relief that their own fortunes do not rest on the decisions of the cadres.[5]

From the perspective of students other than the cadres, the operation and maintenance of rules often appears to be the raison d'etre of the school. Faced with a myriad of regulations pertaining to such private behavior as manner of dressing, dormitory conduct and use of alcohol, students often feel that the possibilities for getting into trouble (or failing) are endless. The dominant role accorded to the rules—particularly those governing leisure behavior—is a primary component of student opinion that the school is more concerned with invading the privacy of students than in teaching them something. Implicit in this opinion is the position that students can agree with the formal goals of the school, but not with the latent definition of the nature of students which is built into the school's regulations. Should this ideological discrepancy become apparent in a troublesome way, the student may hear this statement, which often constitutes an administrator's piece de resistance: "If you don't like the way we do things here, you can leave." The difficulties involved in "leaving" a school, or of transferring to another one, are familiar and formidable. Nonetheless, the administrator's point—that the student is expendable, and that the school need not change itself

---

[5] A most striking difference between faculty in the nursing schools which we have observed and faculty in small colleges is the relatively greater autonomy from the administration possessed by the latter. It is noteworthy that the sources for prestige among faculty of nursing schools is sharply limited; here, then, is one possible function of the pressures on academicians to publish . . . their status is less dependent upon recognition by local administrators. The result of the nursing school situation, from the point of view of the students, is a lack of active faculty support in the face of administrators' wrath.

to accommodate her—has been made. These students may form a polar group, in contrast to the cadres; they are overwhelmed by the "stupidity" of the rules; they are singularly impressed with the arbitrariness of the administrators and the vindictiveness of their "goody-good" peers.*

NURSING SCHOOL: THE RULES AND THE STUDENTS

In this chapter, diverse reactions of one class of students to rules governing the General Hospital School of Nursing are documented. The researcher began to gather her data during the summer of 1964. She lived in the dormitory and participated with the students in a wide gamut of activities such as eating ice cream, going to dinner, drinking beer, visiting and joking. The researcher first was introduced by a nursing instructor to several students who were friends and newly elected school officers. During conversations with these girls and others in their group, it was learned that there was another group of students (referred to as the "wild ones") who generally were regarded by the student officer group as being "the opposite from us." Later, the history of antagonism between the two groups was recounted, and reports on the disapproved activities of the wild ones were provided. One member of the student officer group (referred to by the wild ones as the "goody-goods") who had maintained a friendship of sorts with a member of the wild ones introduced the researcher to that group. After being subjected to much testing, the researcher was finally trusted by the wild ones and subsequently conducted intensive research on that group. Follow-up data were gathered on the same class of girls in the summer of 1965 when they were seniors, and again in 1966. Supplementary information was obtained through conversations and interviews with students of another local, church-affiliated nursing school, which will be referred to hereafter as Church School of Nursing.

In many ways, the complexities of rules, "total person" evaluations and the relationships between a school and its students are exacerbated within the special context of a nursing school. Nursing students are expected to face all manner of human misery and even

---

* That such a group, polar to the "student-officer" group, may be the "in group" is familiar—and a nightmare—to administrators. Should such a group develop, attempts will be made to co-opt them and to channel their leadership abilities into "positive" activities.

death with a measure of professional reserve and control, but their private lives are governed by regulations which deny them that maturity which their professional role assumes.

Contradictory demands placed upon nursing students are most glaring; for example, the students are enjoined to exhibit responsibility on the wards, and yet adhere to ward procedures which a) the students regard as impractical, and b) are *not* followed by practicing nurses. They are told that they must "be mature" and yet submit to blanket regulations concerning their off-duty behavior. In short, they are accorded only a limited and inconsistent adult status.

In the nursing school setting, two separate and somewhat divergent ideological strains feed into the seemingly inconsistent demands placed upon the students. The legendary conception of Florence Nightingale as personalizing traditional Christian morality for females stimulates the impulse of nursing schools to stand as guardians of the girls' virtue; virtue is seen as closely aligned with, if not a prerequisite for, adequate nursing student role performance.[6] Accordingly, it is customary at "capping" or graduation ceremonies for students or graduates to recite the "Nightingale Pledge":

> I solemnly pledge myself before God and in the presence of this assembly:
>
> To pass my life *in purity* and to practice my profession *faithfully*.
>
> I will abstain from whatever is deleterious and mischievous, and will not take or knowingly administer any harmful drug.
>
> I will do all in my power to maintain and elevate the standard of my profession, and will hold in confidence all personal matters committed to my keeping, and all family affairs coming to my knowledge in practice of my profession.
>
> With loyalty will I endeavor to aid the physician in his work, and devote myself to the welfare of those committed to my care. (Italics ours.)

---

[6] Some of the effects of the Florence Nightingale heritage have been examined by Whittaker, E. and Olesen, V., The Faces of Florence Nightingale: Functions of the Heroine Legend in an Occupational Sub-Culture, *Human Organization, 23,* 1964, pp. 123-130.

At the same time, advances in medicine have placed increasing demands on the modern nurse, thus emphasizing the need for training nurses in expertise rather than concentrating on the more private aspects of nursing students' behavior. This orientation toward expertise is encouraged by the determination of nurses themselves to elevate the status of their profession. In nursing schools, however, the ideology of expertise weds itself firmly—although less firmly, perhaps, than formerly—to the traditional orientation; the profession wishes to increase the intellectual capabilities of its members but, at the same time, it does not wish to sacrifice instilling those personal characteristics that it believes to be a part of what is known as a "good nurse."[7] The particular combinations of traditional and expertise orientations vary from school to school. A student from Church Hospital School of Nursing remarked, "Between God and Florence Nightingale, we can't do *anything* right." Another nursing student from that same school volunteered, "Besides, it's all such a sham; Florence Nightingale died of syphilis, we *all* know *that*."

The feeling that one "can't do anything right" is, to say the least, an unpleasant one. Although such a feeling may result only partially from established regulations (and partially from the attitudes one perceives those in authority to have), the regulations may lend themselves to this kind of interpretation. As in many other schools, the rules at the General Hospital School of Nursing were, to a great extent, incorporated into the "Student Handbook." This handbook contained specific rules concerning proper attire ("short-shorts" were forbidden), cafeteria hours, and the use of all such facilities as kitchens, the sewing machine, washing machine and the bicycles. The same handbook included grading policies, admission requirements and library rules. The ultimate sanction available to the school was its power to expel deviants, and this topic was treated under the title of "Termination."

The faculty reserves the right to terminate the student's enrollment in the School at any time if the student's personality, conduct, health or level of achievement makes it seem inadvisable

---

[7] For a book-length account of different orientations in the nursing field, see Habenstein, Robert W. and Christ, Edwin A., *Professionalizer, Traditionalizer, and Utilizer*, University of Missouri, Columbia, Missouri, 1955.

that she should continue in the School. Fees will not be refunded.

Students are forbidden to bring full, partially full, or empty liquor bottles into the Nurses' Residence. Any student found possessing the above materials will be brought before the Advisory Board of the Student Council and will be subject to expulsion from the School.

These two paragraphs were the complete "Termination" section. The prominent position accorded the rule against drinking alcoholic beverages is common in small schools generally, not just nursing schools. The inclusion of a rule concerning empty bottles in General's set of regulations was stimulated by reports that the wild ones had "emptied" bottles during a birthday party held in the dormitory. Thus, to protect the rule prohibiting drinking in the dormitory, the ancillary rule prohibiting *bottles* was invoked.

A student could also be asked to withdraw from General Hospital School of Nursing should she fail to maintain a grade of 75 in any subject, or should three of her clinic instructors report her ward performance to be unsatisfactory. These avenues of failure were discussed in the handbook, under the title of "Withdrawal." In reality, however, both the academic and clinical evaluations of the students were influenced by individual, personal factors. Some girls commented on instructors who had been "particularly helpful" to them in classes, and the handbook itself stipulates that "Grades are based on comparison of performance within the same group and on achievement at the present level of performance and not as an accomplished practitioner." More pointedly, the philosophy that each student's performance should be evaluated individually is espoused throughout the handbook, and the reports of the girls indicated that, most assuredly, this was the means by which individuals were encouraged to withdraw from school, or were assisted to remain. In sum, students were not evaluated in a universalistic manner either in their classroom and ward performances or in their deviance and conformity with respect to the rules governing leisure behavior, even when the crucial issue of expulsion was involved. The student may or may not have done well academically and may or may not have followed the rules; the important thing was whether a total evaluation resulted in the administration's opinion that she was, in some way, "not suited for nursing."

Our purpose is not to decry the intrusion of "personal" factors into a potentially impersonal situation. Rather, we should like to point out that it is the blurring of whim and predictability by the evaluators—in their employment of personal considerations—which stimulates the antagonism and frustration of the students. Thus, a student from General Hospital School of Nursing offered: "They've (the administration) just been waiting to catch me on something they can kick me out for, for years." And, a student of Church Hospital School of Nursing complained, "They're (the administration) so *irrational;* you absolutely never know how they're going to react to *anything.*"

Several students at General reported that the basis for determining "whether or not you're punished is who you are, not what you've done." A primary component, then, of individualized punishment was a girl's "reputation." And many students expressed the opinion that the content of one's reputation did not hinge primarily upon one's class or ward performance, but rather consisted chiefly of how one behaved during leisure hours. Although administrators seldom would admit to the operation of such subjective evaluations, one administrator at General offered the following summary explanation for asking a girl to withdraw: "She just couldn't accept (those in) authority." Often, too, a student's reputation was established through the friendship group to which she belonged—one is "known by the company one keeps."

Our observations revealed that the class in our sample was divided into nine rather discreet friendship groups. Circles of friends would eat meals, visit and engage in a variety of leisure activities together, although some degree of contact would be maintained with girls outside their group. The girls themselves reported that their class was "real cliquish."

To obtain more precise information concerning the existence and memberships of the groups, the researcher (with some assistance from three class members) compiled a tentative listing which separated all members of the class into the friendship groups to which they appeared to belong. Two respondents from each group were then asked to evaluate the listing and make any changes which they believed would improve its accuracy. The 18 respondents suggested a few actual membership changes and a great deal of information was obtained concerning the history of a girl's group membership and her status within the friendship group. Each respondent was also asked to rank the nine friendship groups according to the degree to which "the administration would approve/disapprove of their behavior if the administration *really knew* what was going on."

All respondents listed the wild ones as the group whose behavior would be the *least* acceptable to the administration, and 13 of the 18 respondents ranked the goody-good group as being the one whose behavior would be the *most* acceptable to the school administration. (Similarly, an administrator warned that it would be difficult to secure the cooperation of the wild ones for the research, and arranged for the researcher to be introduced to the student-officer group first to provide entry into the entire class.) Upon questioning, the respondents offered a variety of reasons for their choices, but generally included the opinion that the wild ones broke the rules, and didn't exhibit the "right kind of attitude toward the school; they seem to be against *everything.*" The goody-goods, on the other hand, "seem to be ideal; they hold offices, and seem to be at ease with the instructors." One girl observed that "they (the student-officer group) are even all *blondes.*" Another girl, when questioned concerning why she had put these two particular groups in opposite positions, answered, "Well, it just seems like the one group *makes* the rules and the other group *breaks* them."

THE GOODY-GOODS

The goody-goods often would *separate* and go to their individual rooms to sleep during the hour and a half (or two hours, depending upon individual work and class schedules) free time between getting off duty and going to dinner in the hospital cafeteria. If one girl had received a gift from a patient or the patient's relatives during the day, or had received interesting news in the mail that afternoon, she would share that event with her friends. Much of the discussion centered on such personal events. Such interaction would customarily take place twice and in two different locations—a room on the fifth floor and one on the sixth.

Occasionally, one or two would sunbathe during that period, and twice the two student leaders met privately to make plans for the first student-body meeting at which they were to preside. Usually, however, short exchanges in which the girls inquired about each other's days and received replies indicating that nothing significant had occurred, were followed by the girls' going to their rooms and sleeping, reading their mail, and then preparing to go to dinner.

This group often went to dinner in "shifts," and if no places were available, the late-comers would sit at another table in the dining room. The important thing, though, was that a member of this group did not go to dinner early by herself. On those occasions on which a group member went to dinner late, she would join members of her own group, if she could.

When, after much planning, the group cooked a meal in the dormitory kitchen, all members were included; only if a member had a dinner date would she be absent. The group did not cook more than once every two weeks, however, and these occasions were generally "timed" so that all members could attend.

Because four of the eight group members were engaged by the summer of 1964, and two of the remaining four were to be engaged soon, members of this group dated frequently. Due to their engagement or near-engagement status, the group conversations did not revolve around getting dates or gossiping about the dates they'd had, or making plans to arrange dates for others.

None of this group smoked and, although three members drank liquor, that information, obtained during a group interview, was not known by all members of the group. Two of the non-drinkers were surprised to learn that any of their number indulged. Drinking, then, was not a group activity, was not regularly engaged in with other group members, and was not a topic of conversation (with respect to themselves). Except for one member, the group reported that they went to church "pretty regularly" with two of the members going to church often and together.

The girls often visited each other's homes on weekends; this occurred primarily among three girls whose homes were in the same area. A major activity during the week, then, was anticipating or reporting weekend experiences. The student-officer group was a quiet one, seldom making noise by laughing or talking loudly. The girls spent much time polishing their shoes, cleaning their dormitory rooms, and assuming the complex duties of school officers and friends of officers.

The primary function of these student officers (*as* student officers) was to mediate between the students and the administration. In large part, they communicated suggestions *which originated in the administration* for altering rules or school policies. The amount of change which originated with the students and was an expression of their will was minimal. The officers explained this situation in terms of student apathy. The question, of course, is whether student apathy stimulated administrative domination of student government or vice versa. Although the goody-goods preferred to think that the former was the case, they provided no evidence that they, as enlightened student officers, could instigate any real changes in the nursing school. Since they represented the "establishment," so to speak, it is not likely that they would have wanted to instigate changes in the first place.*

THE WILD ONES

The wild ones, those who received every possible vote as being the group whose behavior would be the *least* acceptable to the administration, preferred to call themselves "the non-conformists." This group consisted of six members, one of whom was a freshman. The inclusion of a freshman was, in itself, deviant, as all other groups were segregated along class lines. The members of this group all lived on the sixth floor in one wing of the dormitory, their rooms being separated from those of the sixth floor division of the student-leader group by a long corridor.

The wild ones traveled together as a single unit, once the separation dictated by the work day was over. With the rather frequent exception of one girl (who was excluded from the group, by the summer of 1965) they regularly met in one of the dorm rooms after work and discussed what kinds of activities they might engage in that evening. They would also recall funny or irritating experiences of the day, and reminisce—mainly through jokes—about parties and events which they had enjoyed or suffered in the past. One of the major descriptive characteristics of this group was that they laughed a lot and were noisy.

Their rooms were unusually messy, and the members sat or lay on the bed of the room being used. When the bed space was taken, they would lie or sprawl on the clothes on the floor or on the one chair. There were two subdivisions within this group, each consisting of three members. Their rooms were at opposite ends of the dormitory wing. The group meetings occurred in rooms belonging to the subdivision that included the freshman, although two of the

---

* A powerful device for controlling possible innovations stimulated by students was utilized by Church Hospital School of Nursing. There, no class meetings were allowed, except in the presence of the (faculty) class sponsor.

three girls in the other subdivision shared a room, and had much more space in which to entertain.

The jokes and conversation of this group were braced by swearing. The customary word used in referring to a non-group member was "bitch." This appellation was extended to teachers, administrative officials, doctors, and any one else who had caused discomfort or restriction for any member of the group.

As in the student-leader group, their favorite group activity, while in the dormitory, was visiting with each other. They tended to reminisce about group, rather than individual, experiences; funny aspects of parties they had attended, or difficult situations involving school officials, proprietors of motels, or dates would be recounted, with every phrase stimulating a series of memories for each girl, and making the entire group laugh. The laughter would subside, then some member would make another remark, and the process would be repeated. The number of times the "phrase-laugh" couplet would recur depended upon many things—whether or not the phone rang, whether or not a non-member "intruded," and whether or not a member wanted to introduce another subject (often a complaint about something). Barring such interruptions, these sessions could easily continue for half an hour.

No member of this group was engaged. A great portion of their time was spent in trying to get dates, talking about fellows previously dated, and planning parties. The party planning activities were concerned primarily with liquor, for the chief mechanism of the group's self-identity of being "deviant" was that the group members all drank a lot. It should be noted, however, that although the identity of "heavy drinkers" was one of great importance to members of this group, they did not, in fact, drink much. Many evenings two of the girls would have nothing alcoholic to drink and the others would have no more than two drinks. The "heavy" drinking took place at parties when at least one or two girls would get drunk, act up, get sick and then retire for the evening. Another point of pride, fun and identity for this group was that they went to bars which were frowned upon, if not actually "off limits," according to the rules. Almost every evening, those members of the group who did not have dates (generally four of them) would return to the dorm following dinner, change clothes, and go to their favorite bar "hangout." The owner welcomed them and often gave them free beverages when they arrived and money to play the juke box.

His friendliness and generosity were explained to the researcher as being the result of the girls being "good for his business," because "last year, this place was really jumping." The girls would proceed to dance with each other, offering suggestive modifications of such standard dances as the twist, dog or swim. These performances were appreciated by the other patrons of the bar, usually all men, and this appreciation was presumably the reason for their buying drinks for the girls. Also, the men would come to the girls' table, visit, and be well received until some type of impropriety or pushiness occurred; the girls wanted to have fun, but they had no intention of tolerating vulgar conversation. A man also would be given the impression that it was time for him to leave if he stayed after the first drinks he had purchased for the girls were consumed and did not offer to buy more. Remarks and witticisms would be exchanged with the male patrons who were seated at the bar or at other tables. This meant that the conversation often became quite loud, as did the laughter. It also meant that the patrons of the bar were becoming "organized" around the group of girls, and that the girls would remain the center of attraction, whether or not they continued to dance.

According to the girls, however, their past experiences in the bar were far more enjoyable than the present ones; they reported that they had slowed down quite a bit in this bar because they were afraid the school administration "would find out and would kick them out of school." "If we were really doing something *wrong*, it would be different." "Hell, *anything we* do, is wrong." "If you listen to the rumors, there's *nothing* we haven't done . . . we were even prostitutes at the Bat (a hotel in the area)." "They (the administration) actually had people *spying* on us; of course, most of those brown noses were only too happy to do it."

The girls in this group often went home on weekends, but the weekends which were most anticipated were those during which parties were to be held. The girls would save their allowances, do baby-sitting and cut down on other expenditures, in order to rent a motel room for one or both nights of the weekend. Very often their liquor, as well as some of the money required for the room, would be furnished by the mother of one of the girls.

The wild ones spent very little time alone. Group membership seemed to carry with it the obligation (as well as perhaps the desire) to be with the group. The joking system was elaborate, as has been mentioned, and an outsider found it difficult to discover why they were laughing, or what was going on. The wild ones did not welcome visitors to their get-togethers; they thrived on secrets, and an outsider posed the threat of "carrying tales" or of getting them into trouble.

In summary, whereas the student-officer group was noticeably quiet and did not use swearing, the wild ones were notoriously loud and used swearing as a form of humor and communication, as well as to express hostility. The student-leader group went home every weekend; whenever possible, the wild ones went to a motel for partying. The most discriminating index of the differences between the two groups, however, centered on their reactions to the rules.

THE RULE-MAKERS VS. THE RULE-BREAKERS

Many practices of the wild ones were, of course, either explicitly against the rules of the school, or would certainly have been frowned upon—according to the girls—if the school administration had known about them. On one occasion, one of the girls stated that the rules of the dormitory and of the school "don't really bother us a hell of a lot," and "Hell, I'm *glad* we have to get in at a decent hour . . . otherwise, I'd *never* get any sleep." At the same time, the girls did not want the rules to "get in our way" or interfere with "what we want to do." If a rule *did* happen to prohibit what the girls wanted to do, it would not only be disregarded or circumvented, but would be despised and bitterly condemned as well. It was not merely the content of the rules which concerned the group, but also the "nerviness" or presumptuousness of those who made the rules. Although the wild ones felt a great deal of anxiety concerning whether or not they'd be "kicked out" because they broke rules, they nonetheless protested: "They (the administration) make such a big hairy deal out of everything! The littlest thing, and they're ready to have a coronary."

Conversely, during the period of time the researcher spent with the goody-goods, *no* comments were made by the group members which were critical of the rules. None of the references they made to rules could be construed to indicate that they believed any rule to be questionable. On one occasion, for example, the girls told the researcher that she could not go to the hospital cafeteria wearing shorts because no one was allowed in the dining room unless wearing a skirt. This statement was followed by no explanation and no remarks, positive or negative; it was a simple fact of life which would, presumably, gear one's behavior.

During the month of July (1964) a student-body meeting was held. The two newly elected officers from the student-officer group presided. One of the major reasons for calling the meeting was to take a vote concerning adding a rule which would make it necessary for girls to be dressed when they went to get candy from the machines in the basement in the evenings. The student leaders were in favor of the additional rule, which would facilitate allowing girls and their dates to use the basement "rec room" in the evening. After minimal debate and minimal interest was expressed, the new rule was passed. The student officers emphasized that the proposed rule had already been discussed with the administration and that the administration was "in favor," although the head of the nursing school had stated that it was "up to the girls."

While the two members of the student-officer group were directing the meeting, the deviant group was involved in conveying the impression that they were disinterested in the meeting and its proceedings. This impression was not conveyed just to each other, but also to members of other groups. They set each other's hair, pretended to doze, and yawned when someone made a point either in favor of or opposing the proposed rule. When the time came to vote, they made a production of voting twice by raising their arms half-way for both *pro* and *con* the rule. Their opinion of the entire student-body organization was that "Miss X (the nursing school director) runs this place," and "this student government is just a figurehead deal—a rubber stamp for Miss X." They all thought it was terribly funny that whether or not to "dress" to go down to the candy machine would become a big issue. This, as usual, stimulated a joke as one girl remarked, "Hell, they're all as fat as I am. They don't need the candy, anyway." The student-leader group viewed its position as rule-makers with no little amount of seriousness; the wild ones considered that process as being a "sham" and lavished the entire student-government effort with derision.

During the summer of 1964 a new food rule, which was to take effect early in the fall, was instituted. This rule limited the amount of food each girl would be allowed to take from the cafeteria. The different responses to the announcement of this additional regulation provide a good index of the differences between the two groups, with respect to their views of the administration's influence on their lives. This rule stimulated little reaction from the goody-goods; one member noted that "Some girls really overdo it, and take much more than they even want." Another observed, "There's really an awful lot of waste." Other than this exchange of comments, the group did not concern itself with the rule, one way or the other. In short, it was perceived to be a legitimate control, and one which would not really alter the group's food-taking activities.

The wild ones, however, attacked the rule with great gusto. They were affronted. What business do *they* have telling us how much we can eat?" "I'd like to see X (the school administrator) live on that amount of food. Hell, she probably eats that much for breakfast." "It isn't enough that we have to pay to *work* here (referring to the services provided on the wards by student nurses), but now they don't even want to *feed us*." "Well, we still have the rest of the summer; let's hog (waste) as much food as we can." Thus, the wild ones did not evaluate the rule in terms of what might have stimulated it—as was the case with the student-leader group—or only in terms of the effect it might have on the dining-room activities of the group, but as still another encroachment of the administration on their private lives.

JUDGMENTS AND JUDGES

The wild ones repeatedly expressed the wish: "They should judge us on our nursing; that's why we're here." "What we do in our private lives is our own business; it has nothing to do with whether or not we are good nurses." The *danger* the wild ones felt was not the result of their class or ward performances; they maintained pride in their capabilities as nurses. "If only people would judge us on what they *should* judge us on." "We're damn good nurses. We put a little life in the place. Our patients like us, and we make that morgue seem alive." Similarly, not one student respondent offered criticism of the wild ones' *nursing* abilities, although some other members of the class received bitter criticism in that area.

There were differing reactions to the wild ones among the administrators of the school. The head administrator (Miss X) regarded the wild ones as deviant, to be sure, but not impossible to manage: "Oh, we know how to handle such girls; there's a group of rebels in almost every class." That they were, in a sense, part of the school tradition was never communicated to the wild ones. Although they were aware that other deviants had gone before them, the various treatments which had been accorded those institutional ancestors gave the wild ones little comfort. From the wild ones' point of view, the ease with which the administration felt it could handle deviant groups seemed far from routine. Administrative handling of such cases included the option of expulsion, and a former group member had been asked to withdraw during her freshman year.* The remaining group members felt that their own student statuses were in constant jeopardy, partly because of the experience of their friend.

Although the head administrator can be said to have regarded the wild ones with some measure of equanimity, such administrative charity was not extended them from all quarters. The final report of each nursing student is filled out by the assistant head of the school, and remains in the girl's permanent dossier. The final profiles of the wild ones regularly pointed out unflattering characteristics; they were "insensitive to patients," "bossy," "had problems with authority," or were summed up by the cursory and subtly censorious evaluation of being an "average student, average nurse." On the other hand, the goody-goods' virtues were almost without exception extolled in the final report. These girls were "excellent nurses," "understanding," "a good kid," "sincere and considerate." And, of course, their leadership positions were cited as being evidence that an individual was "well accepted," or a "good supporter."†

---

* As is the case with many dropouts, this girl officially left because of academic problems. Nonetheless, she was evaluated by the administration as having "a problem with authority"; the wild ones observed that she had gotten into trouble with the assistant administrator, and *that* was the "real" reason she was "kicked out."

† The average state board examination scores of the goody-goods were only slightly higher than those obtained by the wild ones; certainly, the contrast indicated by the final administrative evaluation was absent. The most striking difference between faculty and administration perceptions of the same student was in the case of a wild one. A faculty member noted that a certain wild one "is able to translate her ideas into action once she is assured that she is not being too 'pushy'." That same girl was described by the assistant administrator as being "bossy" and a girl with "many problems with authority." It is significant, too, that there were no reports concerning problems

The wild ones seemed faintly obsessed with the ironies of their situation: "Wouldn't that be a bitch—to come this far and then get kicked out for something that isn't even any of their business?" Various opinions were expressed concerning why they had *not* been expelled: "If they didn't need their slave labor so much in that damned hospital, we'd *all* be out on our asses." Other tentative explanations of administrative tolerance for them included the possibility that Miss X was aware of the fact that they were good nurses, and for that reason allowed them to remain in school. More frequently, however, the explanations were of the order that "maybe she (Miss X) was wild when she was young," or "maybe she doesn't know," and finally, "yes, she knows but she doesn't give a damn; she's letting us get through anyway."

POSTSCRIPTS

Regardless of *why* the wild ones were not expelled, and regardless of the fact that they were not asked to leave, they did function somewhat as negative role models for their student-nurse peers. Here, the observations of Kai T. Erikson are appropriate. He has noted that behavior (or individuals) labeled as deviant function as boundaries for the social system in which the deviance occurs. Deviance throws into bas-relief the modes of behavior which are accepted, and the individuals who are acceptable, in a given social system. Erikson states:

> . . . and like an article of common law, the norm retains its validity only if it is regularly used as a basis for judgment. Each time the group censures some act of deviation, then, it sharpens the authority of the violated norm and declares again where the boundaries of the group are located.[8]

with authority on the job, or in working with the physicians; apparently any trouble the girls had with authority was restricted to the authority of the administration. Further, it might be argued that it is an *empirical* question whether the "problem with authority" was the student's problem, or that of the administrator who seemed to perceive it as a particular pervasive difficulty.

[8] Erikson, Kai T., Notes on the Sociology of Deviance, in Becker, Howard S. (Ed.), *The Other Side: Perspectives on Deviance*, The Free Press, Glencoe, Illinois, 1964, p. 14.

It is significant that not all norms serve to separate "we" from "they," or to discriminate between the approved and disapproved categories of individuals. Only certain norms are so constituted and so emphasized as to perform such functions. Certainly, the decision of what behavior to punish is not made according to random criteria. Given that not all norms or rules are enforced, and that not all are enforced to the same degree, the norms which become issues may be regarded as a special type. Erikson's theory addresses itself to community boundaries and formal institutions such as prisons or mental hospitals which are designed to segregate official deviants. In part, complementary theoretical positions are suggested by the settings we have described.

We have noted that an important component of the complex system of social control effected by the General Hospital School of Nursing was the student-leader group. More than the mutual antagonism felt by the wild ones and the goody-goods bound the two groups together. They were linked as "opposites" by administrators and peers alike. The "paired-opposites" treatment of the goody-goods and the wild ones suggests that individuals who are regarded as deviant with respect to institutionally specific rules, or with respect to diffuse mandates, are not so labeled as a result of the application of such formal criteria exclusively. Individuals may also be regarded as deviant when they enact behavior patterns, or express attitudes, which are somewhat *archetypical* of the norms. Thus, the "personalized" component of the social system described herein means, in part, that *people* evaluate, reward and punish *people*. The school administrators, for example, used students, and to a large extent these two groups from the same class, as comparisons for each other.

From this view, the cadres help determine the boundaries of the social system, as much as do the deviants, and not only because conformists perpetuate traditional norms. Cadres also may encourage the re-emergence of established but relatively inactive norms and may, in fact, be instrumental in the formulation of new rules.[9]

---

[9] Bendix and Berger, in "Images and Concept Formation," suggest that both boundary-extending as well as boundary-maintaining activities of individuals must be examined. It is probably the fact that systems tend to react to boundary-extension by increased efforts of boundary-maintenance at precisely those points that contribute to the "Saints and Sinners" notion of Parsons, and the hair's breadth

Thus, if deviants are to be identified in terms of their function of establishing boundaries, the goody-goods are as deviant as the wild ones. Under any label, however, those students who are perceived as the embodiment of the normative *ideal* often put the teeth into the treatment accorded those who violate the norms, as much as those perceived as violating the norms etch more clearly those individuals who seem to fly high within the organizational system.

The case of the wild ones of General Hospital School of Nursing goes beyond Erikson's point that deviance *establishes* the boundaries of a social system. Rather, the wild ones offer evidence that institutional deviance may result from a dispute concerning where those system boundaries are to lie. The wild ones disagreed that the school's territory, i.e., the range of behavior subject to its control, extended into their private lives. They felt that the authority of the school should be addressed primarily to areas of nursing expertise rather than to questions of morality or off-duty behavior. It is in this sense that the wild ones can be described as having been engaged in a struggle to maintain (or establish) personal autonomy.

Upon graduation, the formal evaluations of this class of students were drastically altered. No longer were the girls' private lives construed to have such important bearing on their expertise as nurses. To be sure the school "let them (the wild ones) get through." It is noteworthy, however, that all except one of the wild ones became employees of General Hospital after their graduation. Clearly, the dissatisfaction they felt for the school while students was not generalized into dissatisfaction with their nursing experiences in the hospital. Indeed, by their senior year, the wild ones had established close relationships with the doctors and loyalty toward General Hospital itself had supplanted much of the antagonism felt for the school. Conversely, only *one* of the goody-good graduates was employed by General Hospital. At this point, the irony may lie on the side of the administrators, as the favored students depart for employment elsewhere and the wild ones remain in hospital nursing. The argument that conformity to rules governing leisure behavior and the exhibition of the "right" attitudes toward administrators has little to do with being a practicing nurse, gains considerable

---

difference between "Heroes and Heretics." Bendix and Berger's discussion is in *Symposium on Sociological Theory,* Gross, L. (Ed.), Harper and Row, New York, 1959, pp. 92-101.

respectability and suggests that such attributes may constitute the earmarks of a good *student* nurse only. While those same individuals were students, however, the stigma of being a rule-breaker or the encomium of being a rule-maker was a very real thing.

A crucial question emerges from these observations: To what extent are "total person" evaluations necessary or even desirable in settings such as that of the General Hospital School of Nursing? In what ways is it desirable and possible to reduce the degree of "total institution" character of schools which so often draws the attention of all from the formal goal of the institution? To that end, several structural changes in diploma schools comparable to General Hospital School of Nursing may be in order. These are discussed in Chapter 7.

It is well known that the problems of administrators are many, and few people could escape having sympathy for one in that capacity; it is our position, however, that the problems of *students* in "idyllic small schools" boasting individualized treatment have gone largely unnoticed. Perhaps we have heard enough of the "administration's point of view;" perhaps we have thought too little about what parts of the system—perpetuated and developed by administrators—might be eliminated or altered for the benefit of students other than the cadres. Some action in this direction may well be required before successful completion of a nursing education program will begin to connote the acquisition of skill and knowledge, rather than merely being evidence of one's ability to "play the game."

Chapter 7

Implications and Recommendations

This concluding chapter summarizes what appear to us to be the key problems of the diploma schools of nursing as revealed by our study of a particular school. Although we have focused on the diploma program, the implications of our findings have relevance for all types of nursing education programs, particularly those in junior colleges or those which involve close affiliation between diploma schools and junior colleges.

The major problems confronting diploma schools of nursing, as we see them, can be listed and defined as follows:

1. *Recruitment*

The attraction of students of adequate intellectual and motivational levels who plan to remain in nursing on the completion of their training as well as after marriage.

2. *Retention*

The reduction of the dropout rate by modifying those institutional factors that contribute to or maintain a high rate of loss.

3. *Socialization*

The training of students so that their image of nursing and the personality characteristics they develop are consistent with high levels of performance in the nursing role and reflect institutionalized values generally held in society for nurses.

4. Organizational Structure

The revision of school rules and regulations, and the reduction of a "total institution" environment in order that educational functions would be separated from other functions.

RECRUITMENT

Students entering the diploma schools of nursing are not usually among the highest ranking graduates of their high-school classes, nor is their academic interest and motivation high compared with that of students entering college. Instead, they have a strong interest in helping others and a practical vocational rather than professional career orientation. The academic content of courses does not attract or stimulate them. The challenge of nursing is in the clinical setting rather than the classroom. Recruitment appeals which are based on altruistic motivations and even the "selfish" motivation of receiving gratification from helping others, are more likely to appeal to these girls than those stressing a career orientation or intellectual challenge.[1]

They come mostly from the lower middle-class segment of the population with some small proportion coming from families in which the father is a professional person and the mother is a college graduate. The girls from higher social class levels tend to be lower ranking students, however, so that the over-all picture of lower academic and intellectual motivation remains. The not-so-bright girls from wealthier families often show an ability to succeed in nursing school above that which would be predicted for them on the basis of their high-school performance and are comparatively more likely to complete the program; these girls represent a sounder investment for the school than the low-ability, low social-class student. Nursing could be made to represent a desirable and attractive alternative to these girls who, because they are not outstanding

---

[1] Bressler and Kephart make a similar recommendation when they report that a "high percentage of nurses . . . found that 'altruistic' satisfactions provided the single greatest source of gratification in nursing." Bressler, M. and Kephart, W., *Career Dynamics*, Pennsylvania Nurses Association, Harrisburg, Pennsylvania, 1955.

in their academic performance, are not interested in or eligible to enter college. Recruitment appeals that are directed specifically to these girls and which would attract more of them to nursing could stress that nursing offers: 1) some advanced education; 2) a "degree" equivalent in the R.N.; 3) opportunity to travel; 4) preparation for employment; and 5) improved chances to marry into a higher social-class level than their own.

Given these characteristics of entering students, increasing or raising academic requirements and standards is likely to produce problems for the diploma schools. Since the students are not usually academically oriented or motivated, raising standards could have the effect of increasing the dropout rate. What seems to be necessary is for the schools to capitalize on the fact that entering students are interested in nursing *practice,* not theory. Academic requirements serve to discourage some students. This does not mean that standards should be lowered. However, it should be possible for the curriculum to achieve a better integration of academic content and clinical practice so that the entering student's initial high interest in participating in nursing activities can be maintained, and to build from this interest into the more academic and theoretical aspects of nursing. At the present, many curriculum plans assume that stimulation and interest can be enhanced by first exposing the student to academic content and impressing her with the importance of knowing theory and general principles. Our suggestion is to reduce the initial heavy academic load in the first year and capitalize on the high level of motivation to *practice* nursing which entering students have.

The implication of these recommendations for diploma schools, if they continue to draw from the same segment of the population as they are now doing, is that they will have less difficulty in securing affiliation with junior colleges than with senior colleges or universities. If they were to "go collegiate," the chances are that they would be less able to attract students or to retain those that currently are attracted.

It is not possible for all such schools to affiliate with colleges or universities partly because many of their nurse faculty members have no degree beyond the B.S. and there are not enough trained nurses with advanced degrees to staff such an expansion. Incorporation of the nursing school into another educational institution would necessitate a drastic modification of the total curriculum and organizational structure of the school. But, given the fact that there are not enough interested colleges and universities who wish to incorporate these schools, this path is open to only a few. One salutory effect would be that it would remove the nursing school from the domination of the hospital. On the other hand, even collegiate programs are not completely autonomous; their fate may be determined by the university or the university hospital with which they are affiliated.

Affiliation with a junior college holds the greatest promise for the diploma school because junior colleges also draw students from the local area and from the same socioeconomic levels. Their faculties are inclined to be heterogeneous in terms of background and training, do not have a large proportion of doctoral degree holders, and are normally not involved in academic research enterprises or in "publish or perish" contests. Their focus is on teaching and the development of curricula which are structured to meet the needs and interests of the local communities. The level of expectation is more likely to be geared to the local situation than is that of the college or university which draws its students from a national base. For these reasons, affiliation with such institutions, particularly for instruction in the academic areas, e.g., social and biological sciences, appears most promising. As nursing instruction is expanded within the junior colleges themselves, their experience with such programs is likely to suggest new modes of training for nursing and new patterns of inter-organizational relationships.

In 1963, the General Hospital School of Nursing affiliated with a local junior college and contracted for the services of its faculty to teach first-year academic courses. At the same time, it retained its independence by specifying the total curriculum for the nursing program. The junior college developed its own nursing program but the two did not interlock nor were they seen as competing with each other. However, there is every likelihood that they will become competitive as the junior college program expands and as local residents come to realize that it is possible to complete requirements for the R.N. in two rather than three years.* Since both institutions

---

* By 1967, the General Hospital School of Nursing had made plans to shorten the total length of the program to under two and a half years (108 weeks) and to more closely approximate the junior college time schedule. During the first year, students will live in the school

draw from the same segments of the population of the metropolitan area in which they are located, there are added reasons for their being competitive with each other and not with the collegiate schools of nursing.

An additional point regarding recruitment should be noted. The entry of high-school girls into nursing is, for many, an important avenue for social mobility.[2] Girls from families of lower socioeconomic statuses can improve their chances for "marrying up" in the social class system by becoming nurses. We do not refer here to the glamorous and often unrealistic expectation of marrying doctors. In American society women often "marry up" and those who have received some advanced training and professional status are often able to improve their chances for marrying at a higher social level than they otherwise would. Nurses are perceived by society as having acquired a set of skills which have relevance for their maternal and wifely roles. Many girls still retain the notion that nursing is a good preparation for marriage and motherhood.[3] To the extent that this view is accepted in society, men will evaluate nurses more highly than non-nurses when seeking a mate. Girls themselves, and their parents, are aware of these possibilities.

Our data provided some indication that nurses often do "marry

of nursing dormitory but attend classes at the junior college. Discussions and plans for further changes are in progress.

[2] For an elaboration of the relation between occupational choice and characteristics of the female sex role in American society, see Psathas, G., Toward a Theory of Occupational Choice for Women, *Sociology and Social Research, 52,* 1968, pp. 253-268.

[3] Davis *et al.,* remind us that nursing is a "profession that until recently had traded, sometimes overtly, on the dubious and self-effacing appeal of affording young girls excellent preparation for becoming wives and mothers." A professional orientation requires the substitution of this goal but whether social and cultural changes will occur which provide women with a "new, less conflict-laden definition of 'womanly success' . . . and which permit (them) to seriously pursue careers without the fear of completely 'losing out' psychically, if not necessarily materially, on the satisfaction that matrimony and motherhood have afforded women traditionally" remains to be seen. Davis, F., Olesen, V., and Whittaker, E. W., Problems and Issues in Collegiate Nursing Education, in Davis, F. (Ed.), *The Nursing Profession,* John Wiley & Sons, New York, 1966, pp. 174-175.

up." In the first place, a large proportion, 63% of the graduating class, were married or engaged within nine months after graduation.* Of the 49 seniors who graduated in August, 1965, 18 (37%) were married by December. In addition, 2 (4%) were married and 11 (22%) were engaged by the time a follow-up questionnaire was administered in May, 1966, some nine months after graduation. We compared the social class level of the girl (using her father's occupation and education in the index reported in Chapter 3) with that of her husband or fiance and found that, except for two cases for which data were not complete, 58% (18 cases) of the girls moved up one or more levels in social class ranking, 30% (9 cases) stayed at the same level and 6% (2 cases) moved down one or more levels. Of those who moved up, three married or were engaged to a medical student, intern or resident, two to pharmacists and one to a dental student. Of those who stayed at the same level, one was engaged to a resident in the hospital. Twenty-two per cent of those who were married or engaged had found their mates in medical or related fields. There is little doubt that students have romantic notions about marrying doctors as was shown in Chapter 4, and there are enough such instances to support their hopes that this will happen. More realistic, however, is the expectation that the nurse will marry soon after graduation and that her husband will be at the same or higher social class level as her own.

Another aspect of the recruitment problem is the fact that some girls come from small towns to a diploma school located in a city. These girls sometimes have difficulty in adjusting not only to the school situation but to life away from their home communities and families. We have noted earlier (Chapter 3) that some are unable to make the adjustment and drop out of school. Others return to their home communities after graduation and this can be viewed as a loss to the hospital which, after all, would like to graduate nurses who will work there. However, if the school views itself as an educational institution dedicated to the preparation of skilled nurses and the improvement of nurses and nursing, then active recruitment in small towns and places outside the metropolitan area

---

* This rate is close to the rate of 71% married for all women in the United States population in 1960 between the ages of 20-24, an age group similar to that of the graduate nurses in this study. We assumed that the engaged nurses would all marry.

can be undertaken. At the same time, however, the school should make some provision for helping these girls adjust to life away from home and in the city. Recruitment appeals can emphasize the possibilities for entry into the urban and even the national occupational structure, or for placement in the prospective students' home towns. It is possible that a liaison between the hospitals in smaller towns and the diploma schools in the cities could be worked out so that students could be supported by their home hospitals during their training period, and later helped to find employment. The pay-off to local hospitals for providing stipends and assistance for students who may then return there to enter practice in these hospitals cannot be guaranteed, but the costs of such programs would be more easily borne than the cost of supporting their own schools of nursing. Schools that are looking for financial assistance for their students could encourage hospitals to provide scholarships or grants-in-aid in exchange for the promise that the graduate will work in the hospital for a specified time after graduation or, alternatively, pay off the "loan." (Comparable arrangements are made for the training of some other health professionals, e.g., clinical psychologists working for state mental hospitals.)

All of these remarks point up the fact that some diploma school entrants who come from a small community have a local orientation. On the other hand, some of these girls have an orientation toward travel and realize that, because nurses are in high demand all over the country, they can travel[4] and find work almost any place they may choose to go. Recruitment literature and advertisements in nursing periodicals often stress the advantages of life in such attractive places as Miami, San Francisco, Chicago and New York. Various fringe benefits such as residential facilities, swimming pools, and access to resort facilities make the possibility of moving

---

[4] Pape has described the phenomenon of "touristry" as a "form of journeying that depends upon occupation, but only in a secondary sense in that it finances the more primary goal, travel itself." (p. 337). She deals specifically with nurses and notes "these nurses do not follow any orientation to work as a central focus of living; their attention is directed to values outside the job environment and they use their work as a means to other, unrelated ends." (p. 341). Pape, Ruth H., Touristry: A Type of Occupational Mobility, *Social Problems, 11,* 1964, pp. 336-344.

around the country with a group of friends, going from one job to another and "seeing the world" an attractive prospect for girls who "always wanted to get away from home."

The various measures outlined here could be of some help to the nursing schools in attracting students. Further research into the significance of the social class origins and the expectations and motivations of entering students is needed if recruitment is to become more effective in attracting students who have the best chance of successfully completing the program.

RETENTION

How to reduce the dropout rate is a problem for many schools, as was noted in Chapter 3. We believe that, as a result of our study, we can suggest several possible modifications in current procedures that would enable schools to retain and graduate more of their entering students. Perhaps the most crucial of these modifications is the restructuring of curricula so as to make it possible for students to develop a more flexible and individualized program. There should be some arrangement whereby a student who fails a particular course could make it up without having to drop out of school and return the next year. The present curriculum structure adheres rigidly to the cohort or class pattern.[5] Courses are presented in a particular sequence which cannot be varied. For example, the student is ineligible to take Clinical Nursing II unless she has completed certain prerequisite courses. Should she fail one of these prerequisites, she is unable to repeat the course until the following year. This, in effect, means that she must leave school and, should

---

[5] Wheeler describes the pattern in which a group of new recruits enter an organization together and follow a preceding group of recruits in the same institution as a "collective serial" type. In such institutions, individuals are "processed" together but, by virtue of their being with others like themselves, can arrive at "collective solutions to the problems they face." (p. 60). This is also a risk, however, since new recruits may learn from older ones and if things are going badly or morale is low, the preceding class can train the new ones in the prevailing pattern. Wheeler, S., The Structure of Formally Organized Socialization Settings, in Brim, O. G. and Wheeler, S., *Socialization After Childhood,* John Wiley & Sons, New York, 1966, pp. 53-116.

she return the next year, bear the stigma of being a repeater. The cost to the school and the student is unduly severe. This revision is most sorely needed in the curriculum for the first year since it is during this time that most academic failures occur.[6]

The diploma-school model of curriculum structure is different from that found in colleges. Prerequisites and sequences may also exist in college curricula but, particularly in the first year, a student may take a course in either semester. Should he fail it in the first semester, he can take it again the following semester. Largely because the diploma school enrollments and faculties are small, this flexibility is not possible or, at least, is not considered. We suggest that such an arrangement should be worked out. An alternative solution would be affiliation with a junior college, since the semester or quarter system would make it possible for students to begin a course at different times during the year, thereby modifying the cohort or class system. Such a modification would also permit the slower student to proceed at a different pace.

As stated previously, it is ironic that some of the most highly motivated students in the school are those who are in the lowest academic ability levels. With a chance to make up failures or course deficiencies, assistance in the form of counseling, reviewing of course work or tutoring by fellow students, it should be possible for many of these students to "make the grade" in their academic work and go on to become effective practitioners.

Similarly, the school can adapt its procedures so that students who have emotional and personality problems can be helped. Short term treatment or counseling, on either a group or individual basis, can be effective in retaining many of these students. However, such

---

[6] An alternate suggestion by Teal and Fabrizio is that "physiology, chemistry and anatomy courses should receive a thorough revamping to delete non-essential materials to the basic goals of nursing proficiency and other high mortality courses identified by individual schools should receive similar modification." (p. 43). Since the aims of the leaders of the profession are to raise and maintain high academic standards, this proposal is not likely to be adopted. Rather than modify the courses it is possible, as Teal and Fabrizio also suggest, to introduce "how to study courses" to assist all students in meeting the academic requirements. Teal, G. E. and Fabrizio, R. A., *Causes of Student Withdrawal from Nurse Training*, Public Service Research, Inc., Stamford, Connecticut, n. d.

counseling needs to be separated from the academic program of the institution. It cannot be done by one's teachers, the dean, the head of the school or any person who is also in a position to teach or directly supervise the activities of students. Counseling and counselors should be independent of the rest of the structure of the school in order that such services will be utilized by students with the full knowledge that the relationship is confidential and that what they say or report will not be used in making evaluations of their competence as students or nurses. One does not feel comfortable about going to a teacher for assistance with a personal problem; nor, it should be added, are teachers in a school of nursing always competent to provide assistance with the emotional problems that students face.[7] We have noted earlier that the total institutional aspect of the school of nursing produces situations in which the student is constantly being evaluated and judged. This tendency of such institutions makes it even more important that the counseling function be made and kept independent of the evaluation process.

We have noted also that some students are unable to adapt to the demands of a particular institution—they do not "fit." It is not that they cannot make the grade academically, or that they are not motivated to become nurses, but that they may perceive the demands placed upon them as intolerable or undesirable. This is not a cause for alarm unless there are many such misfits in a school. There will always be those who do not like *this* school's routines

---

[7] Teal and Fabrizio recommend that "psychological counseling services be routinely provided to all students, with free access, located to insure privacy and anonymity and with confidential handling of case record files." This recommendation is based on the finding that all students in their study recognized a need for advice and counseling. The type of counseling generally provided was academically oriented rather than therapeutically oriented and was not meeting the personal needs of the non-academic dropout. They also recommend "a general reduction in the tense atmosphere of the nursing education program, increased recreational activities, reduced academic loads during the early periods of training, better living conditions, more counseling services and quicker identification of emotionally oriented individuals . . ." Teal, G. E. and Fabrizio, R. A., *op. cit.,* pp. 42-43.

and procedures but who would enjoy being in *another* school's program. But the "closed" system of education in the diploma schools makes no provision for students to transfer from one school to another and even makes the transfer of credits difficult. More uniformity in curriculum standards would facilitate the transfer of both students and credits and many misfit students could remain in nursing by shifting to an institution more suitable to their particular interests and personalities, not to mention the possibility of transfering for such other reasons as being closer to home.

Finally, an immediate reduction in the number of dropouts (by 25% in this school) could be gained by allowing students to marry and remain in school. Fortunately for the nursing profession, the archaic practice of dismissing students who marry is dying out. It is a commentary on the state of the profession, however, that it has persisted for so long.[8] There has been almost a blindness, among nurse educators, to the fact that marriage is a fact of life and that young girls entering nursing school are very likely to want to marry before they complete the program. Rules requiring the married student to continue to live in the dormitory are ridiculous. Married students could be assisted in finding housing close to the school and hospital so they could continue their studies more easily. The value position that should be adopted is that the student has a right to live a life of her own and if she wishes to marry and attend school, that is her business. She should not need the permission of the school to marry in the first place and she should not be required to live in the dormitory after she is married. She should not be forced to choose between marriage and completing her education. Schools could assist her in finding employment after marriage so that she can remain in hospital nursing, for example, rather than concluding that hospital nursing is not compatible with being a wife and mother. It is likely that if nursing schools adopted a policy of assisting their students who wish to marry while still in school, they would extend such assistance to their graduates also and thereby help to keep them actively employed in nursing.

---

[8] Cunningham has noted that enrollments could possibly be increased by 2,500 if more liberal marriage and residence policies were to be instituted in some 432 schools which still had restrictive rules. Cunningham, Elizabeth V., *Today's Diploma Schools of Nursing*, National League for Nursing, New York, 1963.

SOCIALIZATION

In the process of becoming nurses, the entering students change, as was shown in Chapters 4 and 5, in the images they have of nursing and in their personalities. Our study has not identified the sources of these changes in the personality of the student nurse and it is difficult to know why the personality needs studied change in the way they do. The nursing school experience often has an effect which appears to us to be undesirable, as judged in terms of values which nurses themselves, and society generally, hold for nurses. The significance of these changes for the nursing role requires more direct investigation and research. Exactly how the school could modify its procedures so that students' personalities will become something different from what they are becoming is not immediately clear to us.

Mauksch[9] has described nurses' perceptions of the typical nurse in terms of personality needs similar to those measured by the EPPS. The typical nurse role is seen as one which permits clear, precise, orderly and submissive arrangements of social situations (Deference, Abasement, Order). The nurse is also seen as having very low succorant needs (Succorance), not dependent on others for love, support or protection, and low on sex (Heterosexuality) and emotionality needs. In Mauksch's study, the perception of the typical nurse differed from nurses' self-perception in that higher self scores were obtained on Succorance, Sex and Emotionality. This pattern suggests that nurses negatively evaluate some of the traits which we found to be developing, e.g., Heterosexuality. Mauksch concludes that the pattern in the occupational role shows a theme of internal control with the *typical* nurse being more cautious, less extreme, more controlled than nurses considered themselves to be. These data suggest, says Mauksch, that nursing is seen as a role in which one can meet one's needs to be with people, but in which one also meets one's needs to operate under conditions reinforcing one's proclivity to limited and secure relationships.

The student must adapt to the demands of both the school and hospital. The interests of both institutions seem to be oriented toward the creation of a certain kind of person in a certain role.

---

[9] Mauksch, H. O., The Nurse: A Study in Role Perception, unpublished Ph. D. dissertation, University of Chicago, 1960.

Consequently, the neglect of the person as a person becomes a concomitant. For example, the absence of interest in the individual student, the failure to provide counseling for personality or personal problems, the willingness of the faculty to require that students "shape up" and conform to the demands of the institution, and the labeling of students who do not conform as "troublemakers" all combine to indicate that conformity, within the range of behavior defined by the institution as relevant for student nurses, is demanded. Students learn that they must adapt and function within the defined role. Although some of them indicated to our researcher that they expected to be different or that they would be able to "be themselves" after graduation, the enduring effect of this kind of socialization experience may make such hopes unrealistic. The institutional setting forces the individual to adapt and, as a consequence, to "become" a certain kind of person-in-role. Certainly, the descriptions presented by student nurses of situations in which they find themselves show an increasing callousness and realism, also termed cynicism, in contrast to the idealism with which they entered nursing. We interpreted our data in this area to mean that students adapt to situations *as they find them* and perceive situations as they "really are." As Glaser[10] has put it, "The dilemma for American nursing is that it works in hospitals run by doctors, that it is bound to obey medical orders for the patients' welfare, and that it is a female and less prestigious occupation confronting a male and more respected one." They are pressed into a setting which severely limits the degree of autonomy and control they can exercise.

Nursing students are oriented to "getting through" much as students in other institutions are.[11] What can happen is that the institution eventually "gets through" to the student, i.e., it influences her (or him) to the degree that it makes her into a different person. While the student may think that all she is doing is adapting temporarily in order to "get through," before she knows it, the years have gone by and she has accepted as a necessary fact of life that which she had to do in order to get through. She can then say that

---

[10] Glaser, W. A., Nursing Leadership and Policy: Some Cross-National Comparisons, in Davis, F. (Ed.), *The Nursing Profession,* John Wiley & Sons, New York, 1966, pp. 1-59.

[11] See Becker, H. S. *et al., Boys in White,* University of Chicago Press, Chicago, 1961.

this is reality and that this is the behavior that *must* be performed. Teachers who, when they were in school, said to themselves, "I will only do this now in order to get through" discover later that they require the same things of their students that they resented when they themselves were students. How can such systems be modified or their detrimental effects on the individual be overcome? How can the press of such restraints on personality and perception be changed? Such changes are effected only with great difficulty and with hardly any possibility of making provisions for the student to operate solely as an individual within the total structure. We cannot, as a result of our research, propose to the nursing student that she be more resistant to the demands of the institution. We realize that she is in a relatively powerless position in the institution and that this *is* a fact of life. We can, however, suggest that administrations recognize the need for students to be given more autonomy and a greater sense of control than they now enjoy. It is difficult for those who are in power to extend power to those whom they govern with benevolent intentions, but it is much harder for those who are benevolently governed to demand, as individuals or even as collectivities organized for such a purpose, that rights be extended to them. It is not only desirable that the faculty and administration accord greater rights to students, they have a responsibility to do so. After all, they hope that many of these students will eventually become leaders in the nursing profession. At the same time, the needs of many students for guidance, counseling and a supportive environment as they encounter the strains and anxieties in dealing with human suffering and life-and-death situations must be recognized. The student cannot be left completely on her own. A balance between emotional support for the student and the extension of autonomy in many areas of her life is a goal to be sought.

What model could be presented to the student that will be of greatest value to the profession in the long run? A model, we suggest, which indicates the possibility of change, the inclusion of the rights and concerns of those who are being socialized, the extension of privileges to those on whom the faculty and administration expend their interest and effort. In short, the interests of any professional group can be better served in the long run by including the persons who are being educated for entry into that profession in the process of their own education. This means, in concrete terms, that the student is not to be regarded as a receptacle for knowledge or as a malleable entity to be molded and put into a position, but rather as a functioning person with particular interests and needs that must be recognized and permitted to find expression even at the cost of institutional policy. If such a view is not adopted, the institution we are dealing with is not an educational institution but solely a training school. It becomes concerned only with molding the plastic students who enter the school powerless and who must entrust themselves and their futures to others who "know more than they do and know what's right for them." Given this model, the student, when she becomes a practicing member of the profession or a teacher herself, will know no other model. She will, in turn, say to entering students whom she may supervise on the wards or teach in the classroom, "this is what you must do and this is what you must know and I know what's best for you."

Increasingly, in mid-twentieth century, education is being recognized as a process involving teacher and student in an educational "experience." In colleges and universities teachers are being influenced by students and institutional changes are developing as a result. Student evaluations of teachers and courses provide teachers with feedback from which they can learn much. We do not suggest that such a model can be adopted in its entirety by the school of nursing. We do suggest, however, that the model of education as an experience involving two parties both of whose interests must be recognized and met is a more desirable model for the long-run interests of the profession than the one currently in vogue. The student must be included in the process of her own education in a way that will make her more than a "passive receptacle" of knowledge if she is to become more than merely a performer of a role in the most routine manner.

The routinization of function, the mere "performance of a job," in bureaucratic organizations such as the modern hospital can be an important means of defending the self from the institution. It appears to us that there is a growing tendency for this to happen within the bureaucratic organization of the school of nursing, as is evidenced by the "total institution" aspect of the schools. To change this trend would require that nursing leaders change their philosophies of education. The current ideology of patient-centered care, emphasizing as it does, the interpersonal and psychological aspects of nursing care, could be extended to reorganization of the educational process itself and make both the student and the faculty aware that the resolution of problems of communication and human relations involve structural and organizational changes. The dyadic interpersonal model of human relations is limited in that it fails to recognize the broader institutional contexts in which such relationships exist. There is every reason to expect that students who are presented in nursing school with an ideology that they cannot implement in the hospital will not only be discouraged in entering hospital practice[12] but will also view their education and training experience as not being consistent with the professed ideology. Ideologies such as this, if they are as valuable and desirable as their proponents believe, have to be espoused wholeheartedly and given viable expression in daily interactions involving teacher and student. A patient-centered ideology could be advocated with greater consistency if those who advocate it were to adopt a student-centered educational philosophy.

At the time of our study, this ideology was advocated in the curriculum of the General Hospital School of Nursing but not in the over-all organization of the school. Students were taught the importance of understanding the patient's needs, relating to him as a person, and utilizing all their skills in treating the patient as a whole person rather than as a "case." Yet, in the projective stories written by seniors, we found (Chapter 4) expressions of cynicism or realism which we interpreted as a reflection of their knowledge

---

[12] Davis has noted that the collegiate school graduate shows a rejection of hospital nursing, largely due to the disillusionment over the dichotomy between the school's ideology (which "emphasizes the interpersonal aspects of nurse-patient relations, comprehensive approaches to nursing care, health teaching, and a problem-solving stance toward issues of patient care") (p. 164), and the reality of everyday hospital nursing ("the bureaucratic depersonalization of the patient, the failure to extend emotional support, the obsessive concern with technical procedures to the detriment of psychological welfare") (p. 165). As Davis concludes, "rather than firing the students with reformistic zeal, the net effect of the ideology is to dissuade large numbers of them from working in hospitals once they graduate. The question remains as to whether collegiate schools can long function as a viable professional force if the doctrines they propagate serve, even unwittingly, to drive away so large a segment of graduates from the core work locale of the profession." (p. 167). Davis, F., Olesen, V., and Whittaker, E. W., *op. cit.*

of "the way things are" in a hospital. Seniors perceived things as routine. Patients were not seen as whole persons with distinct personalities. Freshman nursing students, perhaps, reflecting their "book learning" rather than clinical experience, did have such perceptions. If the ideology has already faded among seniors, there is little chance that it will be regained in later years. There is little support for this ideology within the structure of work relationships and hospital organization. However, there is an opportunity for the nursing school to contribute to the advance and support of this ideology by building it into its own structure. That is, were the nursing school to treat student nurses as whole persons, and the faculty to demonstrate concern for the individuals' needs, interpersonal relationship skills could be practiced both in the classroom and on the wards under the supervision of clinical instructors. In many situations involving faculty, administrators and students, effective implementation of this ideology could be fostered. Considerable organizational change would be necessary in order to do this but, if such a re-structuring does not occur, the lesson the student learns is that the ideology is to be embraced intellectually but rejected in practice.

"To practice what is taught" has always been the hardest task that educators have had to face and there is no reason to think it will be easy for nurse educators to begin doing this. To fail to do so, however, will make the teaching continue to appear to be irrelevant and the continuation of present practices the predictable outcome. The new graduate will enter nursing practice seeking an environment in which she can do what she has been taught to value. Failing to find it, she is more likely to leave rather than stay and try to change things because she has never experienced a successful effort to change an organizational structure and is not prepared to do so. Thus, the exodus from hospital nursing may be accentuated by such ideologies, as Davis has noted for collegiate graduates, and the dilemma of nursing education will remain. Junior college programs are not immune from the pattern we have described.

ORGANIZATIONAL STRUCTURE

The imposition of rules on the student body is viewed by the institution as a necessary part of the system. Certainly, it is necessary for schools to have rules and regulations. What we are concerned with is the character of those rules and their consequences as these are related to the aims and goals of the institution. Ideally, rules and regulations should be consistent with the goals of the organization, and should function to achieve, or at least not impede the achievement of, those goals. If, for example, a professed aim of the school is to train nurses of high quality and competence in nursing skills, then evaluation of these abilities and skills should not be influenced by the students' social and recreational activities. Her dating and drinking habits, and her beliefs, values and opinions are, and should be, her own affair. However, the existence of a dormitory run by the school tends to make the private sphere of the student's life, i.e., the after-school and after-work hours, part of the total complex of activities labeled "nursing school." The school thus encroaches upon the student's private, after-hours life. From the school's standpoint, the justification for this, and we must say it is a rationalization rather than an acceptable justification, is that the student is being prepared to enter a profession in which high moral standards are expected. Further, she is entrusted to the care of the institution by her family and, being a minor, must be supervised by a substitute parent. Mauksch[13] also found that the residential arrangements of the nursing school sustain the continuity of controls and common experiences for all students which produces a climate "comparable to that of the army or the convent." The residence is also a source of conflict in that daily work demands require the student to act as an adult when on the ward whereas residence rules and policies are "restrictive and inappropriate."

An easy answer to this criticism would be for the school not to provide dormitory facilities for under-age students. This is too facile an answer; it is probable that dormitory arrangements will continue to be necessary because students are recruited from a wide area and cannot live at home. In addition, many students want the experience of living away from home. The question is, how are they to be supervised and by whom? We recommend that those who supervise the dormitory and after-hours life of the students should not be tied in with the administration or faculty of the school. There may be rules, for example, for times to be in at night, for checking out on weekends, for doing laundry, or for where boyfriends may be entertained, but such rules should apply only to life in the

---

[13] Mauksch, H. O., *op. cit.*

dormitory and infractions should not reflect on or be used in making judgments concerning the performance of the individual in the nursing *school*. It would be conceivable then for someone to be expelled from the dormitory for violating rules concerning hours, but not expelled from school. If such a student were able to provide suitable accommodations for herself outside of the dormitory, and had her parents' consent, she should be able to stay in school. There is no necessity that one live in a dormitory in order to become a nurse, as the junior colleges are proving.

The encroachment by the school into the after-hours life of the student is related to the fact that the dormitory and the school are under the same administration. Furthermore, in the particular instance of the General Hospital School of Nursing, the dormitory is adjacent to the hospital and the classrooms and offices of the faculty are located in the dormitory itself. Thus, it is possible for a student to be seen by faculty at times when she defines herself as not being "on" as a student. One can indeed question whether faculty should be in any position to see how a student behaves during her off-duty time.

The junior college approach to the training of nurses presents an alternative model. It does not provide residential facilities. Students live at home or in places of their own choosing. They are judged on their performance as students in nursing situations and not as rule-abiding dormitory residents. What they do when they leave the classroom and the hospital is not and should not be of concern to the school. Colleges and universities have wrestled with this same problem and have, on occasion, expelled students because of misconduct in the dormitory. We believe that this is a mistake. Unfortunately, there has been a tendency to regard the student status as paramount and to judge all other behavior as relevant to this. As Mauksch[14] notes, the pressure that all behavior be professional and that a nurse is a nurse "completely and all the time" is the most forceful impact of the nursing school.

In this context the question of student government should be considered. If student government is to exist in nursing schools, its provisions for peer group sanctions for institutionally approved or disapproved behavior should not be an extension of a faculty or administrator's point of view. It should not be a "rubber stamp"

---

[14] Mauksch, H. O., *op. cit.*

for the administration but an effective vehicle of student expression. This means that student-government representatives should be included in discussions concerning educational policy and curriculum. The incongruity in student governments lies in the fact that at the same time that students are expected to behave as adults, they are protected, shielded and governed by their elders. Student governments tend to be mere shells which make a mockery of the notion of individual rights and effective expression of student belief. They can be effective only to the extent that their autonomy is real. So long as they represent an extension of the school administration, their officers and their policies will be subject, either formally or informally, to the supervision and approval of the administration. Schools have a real opportunity to present students who are about to enter the world of adulthood with a situation where experimentation and change is possible in a real social system. The learning experiences which can be achieved by making student government truly self-government have not usually been recognized by nursing schools. Experience in running their own affairs could be valuable preparation for the later assumption of administrative roles. The "danger" inherent in extending responsibility and power to student government is that students will make demands and will press for change in the organization of the school, i.e., the status quo will be threatened. This is an almost universal concern among faculties and administrators. It is our contention that the real strength of educational institutions lies in their willingness to develop and experiment with new forms of education. Inclusion of the students in the decision-making process would tap one of the greatest resources of these institutions. It would contribute to the school's ability to adapt to new conditions in an ever-changing society since, by making themselves responsive to the interests of their students, they would be better able to absorb new ideas and, eventually, be more willing to modify prevailing practices. Becker[15] has argued that "reforms in medical education will be most effective when they take into account the collective character of student behavior and recognize the fact that students . . . have a certain degree of autonomy with respect to [academic issues]." This autonomy is based on the development of a student culture in which there is a shared perspective and a sharing of ideas and activities

---

[15] Becker, H. S., *et al.*, *op. cit.*, pp. 438–441.

which are legitimized by that culture. This involvement, which Becker describes, is different from the more organized and institutionally sanctioned involvement, via student government, which we are advocating. It is our opinion that the long-run interests of both students and faculty will be better served by explicit attention to means whereby students are explicitly and directly involved in the affairs of the school rather than relying on the informal structure of the student culture.

Finally, procedures of evaluation which allow faculty and administrators to make judgments and evaluations of students' personalities need to be modified. By adopting a counseling and helping orientation, the school can put itself in the position of trying to maximize the potential of each individual. Rather than adopting some notion of what the ideal personality is and punishing those who do not conform, an alternative approach would seek to discover what is best in each individual and maximize those qualities. A further implication of this approach would be that the faculty itself needs to be evaluated. This is not an argument for student evaluations of faculty and of courses offered, though that is also possible and desirable. It is, instead, a plea for recognition that faculty members also have problems in dealing with students and in making evaluations.

There needs to be some check on the exercise of idiosyncratic and whimsical judgments by individual faculty members. Institutionally, this could be provided by review and evaluation committees which would decide whether students should be advised to withdraw, be placed on probation, or allowed to continue. However, prior to such judgments it would be possible for individual faculty members to exercise their bias in the form of grades. Since these could not be remedied by the student unless appeal or grievance procedures were available, it would need to be recognized that a failing grade in one course represents one instructor's evaluation rather than a damning, global one. Appeal procedures could provide some protection for the student but it would be difficult and embarrassing for a student to initiate an appeal. Evaluation committees could be more effective than they are in assessing the student's academic and clinical performance. An over-all grade average is no substitute for a careful judgment based on clear and well-formulated criteria which are known to students and faculty. Provision should be made for early and regular feedback to the student concerning her performance. Feedback given in a helpful, non-punitive manner would allow her to take steps to modify her behavior, and enable her to grow with greater self-understanding and, at the same time, contribute to a motivation for such growth.[16]

The nursing school faculty is like any other faculty in that its members cannot be regarded as "paragons of virtue" or as ideal persons free from the exercise of whim or bias. Some provision needs to be made for faculty members to obtain assistance in dealing with their own problems, particularly those problems that are manifested in their relationships with students. If there is a spirit of cooperation and helpfulness and an ideology which does more than give lip service to the importance of interpersonal and human relations skills, then the notion that it is only the student that needs help will gradually fade. Both faculty and students need assistance in dealing with problems of learning and living together. Calling attention to such problems can contribute to the overall excellence and quality of the educational institution. Such improvement will eventually be reflected in the quality of the school's graduates.

In conclusion, the problems of the diploma school, as we have noted, include not only those that are unique to such schools, but also many which are generally found in other educational institutions as well. For this reason, we feel that the contributions of this study will be applicable to all types of nursing education programs. Nursing educators and leaders of the profession who are concerned with improving the quality of the education of nurses must face some of the issues that have been presented here. Our hope is that consideration of the issues raised in this study will prove beneficial for students, faculty, administrators, and all who are concerned with improving the quality of nursing and nursing education.

---

[16] Miles has noted that the feedback most helpful for learning is "1) clear and undistorted; 2) comes from trusted, non-threatening sources; 3) follows as closely as possible the behavior to which it is a reaction." Experience accumulated in training groups and in research on the process of individual change supports these conclusions. Miles, M. B., The Training Group, in Bennis, W. G., Benne, K. D., and Chin, R. (Eds.), *The Planning of Change*, Holt, Rinehart and Winston, New York, 1961, pp. 716-725.

Index